Hand-Arm Vibration

DISCLAIMER

The material presented in this book is not intended to represent the only, nor necessarily the best, methods or procedures appropriate for the subject matter discussed, but rather is intended to present an approach, view, statement, or opinion of the authors, which may be helpful or of interest at this time.

Hand-Arm Vibration
A Comprehensive Guide for Occupational Health Professionals

P. L. Pelmear, M.D.
W. Taylor, M.D., D.SC.
D. E. Wasserman, MSEE

VNR VAN NOSTRAND REINHOLD
New York

Library of Congress Catalog Card Number   92-13983
ISBN 0-442-01250-0

Printed in the United States of America.

Van Nostrand Reinhold
115 Fifth Avenue
New York, New York 10003

Chapman and Hall
2-6 Boundary Row
London, SE1 8HN, England

Thomas Nelson Australia
102 Dodds Street
South Melbourne 3205
Victoria, Australia

Nelson Canada
1120 Birchmount Road
Scarborough, Ontario MIK 5G4, Canada

16   15   14   13   12   11   10   9   8   7   6   5   4   3   2   1

Library of Congress Cataloging-in-Publication Data

Hand-arm vibration : a comprehensive guide for occupational health
    professionals / editors, P. L. Pelmear, W. Taylor, D. E. Wasserman.
        p.   cm.
    Includes bibliographical references and index.
    ISBN 0-442-01250-0
    1. Vibration syndrome.   2. Hand—Diseases.   3. Arm—Diseases.
4. Occupational diseases.   I. Pelmear, P. L.   II. Taylor, W.
(William), 1911-   .   III. Wasserman, Donald E.
    [DNLM: 1. Arm Injuries—etiology.   2. Hand Injuries—etiology.
3. Occupational Diseases—prevention & control.   4. Vibration—
adverse effects.   QZ 57 H236]
RC963.5.V5H36   1992
617.5'74044—dc20
DNLM/DLC
for Library of Congress   92-13983
                                                              CIP

"Not only in antiquity but in our own times also laws have been passed in well-ordered cities to secure good conditions for the workers; so it is only right that the art of medicine should contribute its portion for the benefit and relief of those for whom the law has shown such foresight; indeed we ought to show peculiar zeal, though so far we have neglected to do so, in taking precautions for their safety, so that as far as possible they may work at their chosen calling without loss of health. I for one have done all that lay in my power, and have not thought it beneath me to step into workshops of the meaner sort now and again and study the obscure operations of the mechanical arts."

From "De Morbis Artificum Diatriba." Editio Princeps 1700.

Bernardini Rammazzini (1633–1714), Professor of Medicine at Modena and Padua.

Contents

Preface

This book has been written for physicians and other health care professionals. It will also be of interest to allied professional workers as well as lawyers involved in compensation and litigation. It covers the effects of human exposure to hand-arm vibration. It is estimated that hand-arm vibration (HAV) jeopardizes the health and future employability of at least two million workers in the United States and the United Kingdom alone. Such workers are mainly employed in public utilities, manufacturing industry, construction trades, mining, forestry, and agriculture.

A major challenge is the multidisciplinary approach required to evaluate the health effects of vibration since it involves engineering, medicine, physiology, epidemiology, mathematics, and statistics. The current information relating to the hazards, injuries, and disorders of HAV-exposed workers has been extracted from the vast volume of international literature available in these widely differing disciplines.

Despite this wealth of information, gaps exist in the understanding of vibration generation, transmission, and control; the basic physiological response of the blood vessels, nerves, and musculoskeletal tissues to the HAV stimulus; and dose-response relationships. The authors hope that readers will be stimulated by the need for knowledge in this fundamental field where problems can be solved only by combining different disciplines. Further research is needed to evaluate and control the health risks. While more workers are being exposed to HAV, since all countries in the world are demanding greater mechanized production, universally there is an increasing demand for a better quality of life. This book summarizes the present state of knowledge in areas where the authors not only have special interests but considerable personal experience, and sets out preventive and control measures. Hand-arm vibration exposed workers require medical supervision to detect early vibration injuries so as to prevent the serious effects.

The text covers:

1. Health effects of HAV including pathophysiology and epidimiology.
2. Treatment and management.
3. Basic principles and measurement of HAV.
4. Hand-arm vibration standards and guides.
5. Vibration control using engineering and ergonomic principles.
6. Legal and compensation aspects.

Since the terminology of HAV exposure is still evolving, a glossary defining specialized, and often unfamiliar, terms is included. Summaries and literature references are provided for each chapter, and the Appendix contains model health and workplace tool assessment questionnaires.

The contributing editors and authors hope that the historical literature reviews, in addition to up-dates on the medical aspects, will stimulate those willing to advance the medical boundaries of knowledge, and so reduce the disability, impairment, and handicap to workers arising from exposure to HAV.

P. L. Pelmear
W. Taylor
D. E. Wasserman

Contributors

Catherine L. Arkell, LL.B.
Attorney at Law,
Everatt & Co., Solicitors
Evesham, Worcestershire,
WR11 4EU, England.

Thomas J. Armstrong, Ph.D., C.I.H.
Professor, Center for Ergonomics,
University of Michigan,
1205 Beal Avenue, Ann Arbor, Michigan,
48109 U.S.A.

Virginia J. Behrens, M.S.
Epidemiologist, NIOSH,
Cincinnati, Ohio, 45244 U.S.A.

Gösta Gemne, M.D., Ph.D., D.Sc. (physiol)
Associate Professor,
Dept. of Occupational Medicine,
National Institute of Occupational Health,
S-171 84 Solna (Stockholm), Sweden.

David Neusner, LL.B.
Attorney at Law, Embry & Neusner,
P.O. Box 1409, Groton,
Connecticut, 06340, U.S.A.

Peter L. Pelmear, M.D., FFOM., FACOEM.
Consultant, St Michael's Hospital,
Dept. of Occupational & Environmental Medicine,
61 Queen Street, Toronto;
Ontario, M5C 2T2, Canada.

Robert G. Radwin, Ph.D.
Assistant Professor, Dept. of Industrial Engineering,
University of Wisconsin-Madison,
1513 Madison Avenue, Madison,
Wisconsin, 53706 U.S.A.

William Taylor, M.D., D. Sc., F.R.C.P.
Medical Consultant,
Nether Banks, Wick, Caithness,
KW1 5XJ, Scotland, U.K.

Ernst VanBergeijk, B.S.
Ford Motor Co.,
17000 Oakwood Blvd, P.O. Box 1586, Dearborn, Michigan,
48121 U.S.A.

Donald E. Wasserman, BA, MSEE.
Consulting Engineer,
7910 Mitchell Farm Lane, Cincinnati,
Ohio 45242, U.S.A.

1

Anatomy and Physiology of the Upper Limb

P. L. Pelmear

An understanding of the normal anatomy and physiology of the upper limb is necessary for an understanding of the effects of hand–arm vibration (HAV) on the tissues of the upper limb.

ARTERIES

At the outer border of the first rib, the *subclavian* becomes the *axillary artery*. It runs downward and laterally, and terminates at the lower border of the teres major muscle, where it leaves the axilla and becomes the brachial artery (Figure 1-1). The *brachial artery* terminates half an inch below the elbow joint in the midline of the limb by forming the radial and ulnar arteries. The *ulnar artery* passes down the medial side of the forearm. In the upper part of its course it is deeply situated, while near the wrist it becomes comparatively superficial. In addition to giving branches to the neighboring muscles, the ulnar artery gives off recurrent branches from its upper end to the anastomosis around the elbow joint, and small branches from its lower end to the anastomosis around the wrist joint. Its largest branch is the common interosseous artery, which arises in the cubital fossa and, after a short course downward and backward ends by dividing into the anterior and posterior interosseous arteries.

The *radial artery*, arising from the brachial in the cubital fossa, runs downward to the wrist. It is comparatively superficial throughout its whole course, particularly in its lower half. In addition to branches to the neighbouring muscles, a recurrent branch to the anastomosis around the elbow, and a branch to the anastomosis around the wrist joint, the radial artery gives off a superficial palmar branch, which arises just above the wrist and runs down into the hand either through, or superficial to, the muscles of the thenar eminence and may complete the superficial palmar arch.

1

The *superficial palmar arch* is the direct continuation of the ulnar artery into the palm. After crossing in front of the flexor retinaculum, the artery runs downward across the palm immediately behind the palmar aponeurosis. On the lateral side of the palm, it is sometimes completed by union with the superficial palmar branch of the radial artery, but frequently the communication with the radial artery is established through the arterial radialis indicis or the arteries of the thumb. In its course, the arch forms a curve convex downward, the lowest part of the curve lying on a level with the extended thumb. As it crosses the palm, the arch lies on the flexor digiti minimi, the flexor tendons of the fingers and the lumbricals, and the digital branches of the median nerve.

Four digital branches of the superficial palmar arch pass to the fingers. Of these, the most medial runs down the ulnar side of the little finger, and the others pass to the medial three clefts. Each divides into two for the supply of the adjoining borders of two fingers. Each finger therefore receives two arteries on its palmar surface, each derived from a different digital branch. As they leave the arch the digital arteries lie in front of the digital nerves, but they cross one another before reaching the fingers, where the arteries lie posterior to the nerves.

The deep branch of the ulnar artery arises in front of the flexor retinaculum and runs downward and then backward and laterally between the flexor and the abductor digiti minimi muscles to join and complete the *deep palmar arch.*

The radial artery winds around the lateral aspect of the wrist, runs downward over the trapezium and then runs forward and medially between the two heads of the first interosseous muscle. Before it does so, the artery is comparatively superficial, and it gives off a communicating branch to the anastomosis around the wrist and a small dorsal metacarpal branch, which in turn divides into dorsal digital arteries.

On entering the palm, the radial artery at first lies deep to the oblique head of the adductor pollicis muscle. In this position, it gives off the *arteria radialis indicis* and the *arteria princeps pollicis*, which runs downward and laterally on to the palmar surface of the first metacarpal bone and divides into two collateral branches for the thumb.

The direct continuation of the radial artery into the palm constitutes the *deep palmar arch*. It crosses the upper part of the palm in contact posteriorly with the metacarpal bones and interosseous muscles and is related anteriorly to the flexor tendons. It is completed on the medial side by union with the deep branch of the ulnar artery. The arch sends branches upward to communicate with the anastomosis around the wrist, and downward to join the digital branches of the superficial arch at the clefts of the fingers.

Some anatomical variation occurs in 5 percent of subjects, with either the radial or ulnar arteries being absent or unequal in size at the wrist, and the palmer arches may not be complete. In Doppler flow studies, only 9 percent to 11 percent of arches appeared to be incomplete, and in these cases the ulnar artery was usually larger and dominant.

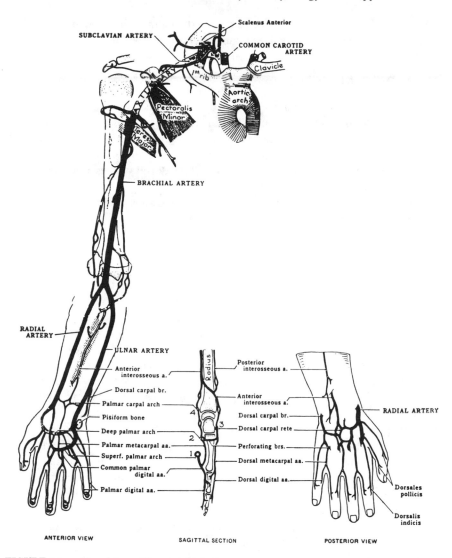

FIGURE 1-1.   Vasculature of the upper limb.

ARTERIOVENOUS ANASTOMOSES

The fingers, in addition to the capillary circulation, contain a number of arteriovenous anastomoses. These are coiled vessels with muscular walls, which are supplied by many nerve endings, but mainly the sympathetic. These arteriovenous shunts are reported to be most numerous in the nail bed, tips of digits, and palmar surface of the digits. Some are also present in the palm of the hand and sole of the foot. These shunts are important in regulating body temperature (see Chapter 4).

SUPERFICIAL VEINS

The *cephalic vein* arises from the radial side of the dorsal venous arch of the hand and ascends to the apex of the cubital fossa. There it receives a tributary from the deep structures of the forearm and gives off the median cubital vein. It then ascends on the lateral side of the biceps muscle.

The *basilic vein* arises from the ulnar side of the dorsal venous arch and ascends up the arm on the medial side of the biceps.

The *median cubital vein* leaves the cephalic at the apex of the cubital fossa and runs upward and medially to join the basilic vein.

FASCIA OF THE HAND

The superficial fascia of the palm of the hand is intersected by numerous fibrous bands that extend between the skin and the deep fascia and is in consequence very tough. The deep fascia of the palmar aspect of the wrist is specially thickened to form the *flexor retinaculum* (transverse carpal ligament), which forms a bridge across the carpus so as to complete an osteo-fascial tunnel for the passage of the flexor tendons of the thumb and fingers. On the medial side, it is attached to the pisiform and the hook of the hamate bones; on the lateral side it is attached to the tubercle of the scaphoid and to the trapezium. Its upper border is continuous with the deep fascia of the front of the forearm, and its lower border blends with the palmar aponeurosis.

Anterior to the retinaculum, the palmaris longus tendon and the ulnar artery and nerve pass into the palm. Behind the retinaculum, within the carpal tunnel, lie the tendons of the flexor pollicis longus, flexor digitorum sublimis and profundus with their synovial sheaths and the median nerve. The lateral attachment of the retinaculum is pierced by the flexor carpi radialis tendon.

The deep fascia of the palm has a very strong central part named the *palmar aponeurosis*, which covers the flexor tendons.

Each finger is provided with an arched fibrous sheath continuous above with the palmar aponeurosis. It is attached to the sides of the phalanges and across the base of the distal phalanx. This fibrous sheath, together with the phalanges and the palmar ligaments of the interphalangal joints, form an osteo-fascial tunnel in which lie the flexor tendons of the finger. It is especially strong opposite the phalanges, but is thin opposite the joints to permit free flexion.

These three structures, the flexor retinaculum, the palmar aponeurosis, and the fibrous flexor sheaths constitute a continuous fibrous sheet whose main function is to hold the tendons in position and so increase the efficiency of the grip.

MUSCLES OF THE HAND

The *lumbrical* muscles arise from the tendons of the flexor digitorum profundus in the palm. They are four in number and each is inserted into the radial side of the dorsal extensor expansion of its own finger. The nerve supply of the lateral two lumbricals is derived from the median nerve while the medial two are supplied by the *ulnar* nerve.

The small muscles of the thumb form the thenar eminence and occupy the lateral part of the palm. The *abductor pollicis brevis* receives its nerve supply from the *median* nerve.

The *flexor pollicis brevis* lies along the ulnar side of the preceding muscle. Its nerve supply comes from the median but it often receives an additional supply from the deep branch of the ulnar nerve and is sometimes solely supplied by it.

The *opponens pollicis muscle* lies deep to the two preceding muscles. Its nerve supply comes from the median nerve. The *adductor pollicis* lies in the lateral part of the palm and consists of two separate heads, the *transverse* and *oblique*. The nerve supply of both muscles is derived from the ulnar nerve.

The *abductor, flexor*, and *opponens digiti minimi* muscles, all receive their nerve supply from the ulnar nerve.

The *interrosseous muscles* comprise four dorsal to abduct the fingers from, and four palmar to adduct the fingers to, the midline of the hand. All receive their nerve supply from the ulnar nerve.

THE BONES OF THE HAND

The carpus consists of eight bones. In the proximal row are the scaphoid, lunate, triquetral, and pisiform bones. The distal row of the carpus consists of the trapezium, the trapezoid, the capitate, and the hamate (Figure 1-2).

THE NERVES

The *brachial plexus* is formed by the anterior primary rami of the fifth, sixth, seventh, and eighth cervical, and the first thoracic nerves together with small communications from the fourth cervical and the second thoracic nerves. The union, separation, and reunion of these nerves in a definite manner constitute the plexus. It commences in the neck and is continued into the axilla (Figure 1-3).

The *median nerve* (C_5, C_6, C_7, C_8, T_1) is closely related to the brachial artery throughout the whole of its course in the arm, and leaves the cubital fossa by passing downward between the muscle bodies. It enters the palm by passing behind the flexor retinaculum. As it lies in the cubital fossa, the median nerve gives off articular twigs to the elbow joint and branches to supply the muscles of the forearm. Within the carpal tunnel, the median nerve divides into lateral and medial divisions.

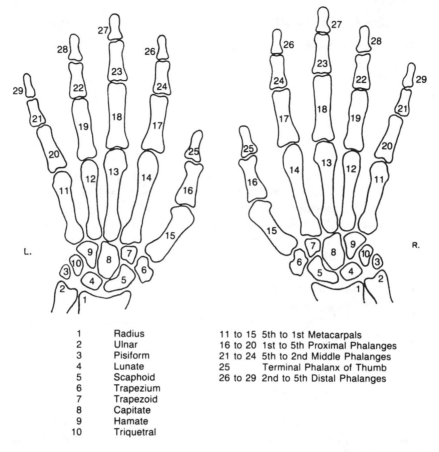

1	Radius	11 to 15	5th to 1st Metacarpals
2	Ulnar	16 to 20	1st to 5th Proximal Phalanges
3	Pisiform	21 to 24	5th to 2nd Middle Phalanges
4	Lunate	25	Terminal Phalanx of Thumb
5	Scaphoid	26 to 29	2nd to 5th Distal Phalanges
6	Trapezium		
7	Trapezoid		
8	Capitate		
9	Hamate		
10	Triquetral		

FIGURE 1-2.   The bones of the hands.

The lateral division gives off, usually by a common trunk, the nerves of supply to the abductor pollicis brevis, the flexor pollicis brevis and the opponens pollicis muscles. It then gives off digital branches to both sides of the palmar aspect of the thumb and to the radial side of the index finger. The last named supplies the first lumbrical muscle. The medial division breaks up into two, and these pass downward behind the superficial palmar arch to the clefts between the index and middle, and the middle and ring fingers. There they divide into collateral branches to supply the adjoining sides of the fingers named. These palmar digital nerves supply not only the whole palmar aspect but also the distal half of the dorsal aspect of each digit. A similar arrangement holds good for the digital branches of the ulnar nerve.

The *ulnar nerve* (C_8, T_1) runs downward on the medial side of the brachial artery. It then crosses the medial ligament of the elbow joint and continues downward to the wrist under cover of muscle. It provides articular branches to the elbow joint,

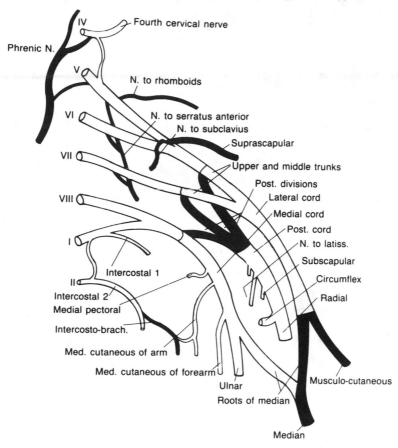

Brachial Plexus

FIGURE 1-3.   The brachial plexus.

muscular branches to the forearm, and palmar and dorsal cutaneous branches. The palmar cutaneous branch is a small nerve that arises in the middle of the forearm and ultimately supplies the skin over the hypothenar eminence. The dorsal cutaneous branch arises about three inches above the wrist and winds around the ulnar border of the forearm and is ultimately distributed on the dorsum of the hand.

The skin of the posterior aspect of the forearm is supplied by the posterior branch of the medial cutaneous nerve (from the medial cord of the brachial plexus) of the forearm along the ulnar border, and by the lateral cutaneous nerve of the forearm along the radial border. A strip of skin down the middle of this surface is supplied by the posterior cutaneous nerve of the forearm (Figure 1-4).

The ulnar nerve enters the palm close to the medial side of the superficial palmar arch. As it crosses the flexor retinaculum it divides into a superficial and a deep

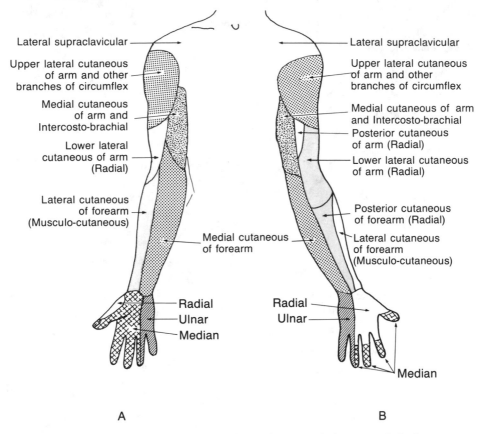

Lateral supraclavicular

Upper lateral cutaneous
of arm and other
branches of circumflex

Medial cutaneous
of arm and
Intercosto-brachial

Lower lateral
cutaneous of arm
(Radial)

Lateral cutaneous
of forearm
(Musculo-cutaneous)

Medial cutaneous
of forearm

Radial
Ulnar
Median

Lateral supraclavicular

Upper lateral cutaneous
of arm and other
branches of circumflex

Medial cutaneous of arm
and Intercosto-brachial

Posterior cutaneous
of arm (Radial)

Lower lateral cutaneous
of arm (Radial)

Posterior cutaneous
of forearm (Radial)

Lateral cutaneous
of forearm
(Musculo-cutaneous)

Radial
Ulnar

Median

A   B

FIGURE 1-4.   Cutaneous nerve distribution of upper limb. A, on the front; B, on the back.

terminal branch. The *superficial terminal branch* divides into a digital branch, which runs downward to supply the ulnar border of the little finger, and a branch that runs down behind the palmar aponeurosis to the cleft between the ring and the little fingers. The latter divides into two branches to supply the adjoining sides of these two fingers.

The *deep terminal branch* turns laterally across the palm and supplies the small muscles of the little finger, the third and fourth lumbricals, all the interossei, and both heads of the adductor of the thumb.

CIRCULATION

The tissues of the body need an adequate blood flow, and to provide this, an adequate head of pressure must be available in the vessels supplying the tissues.

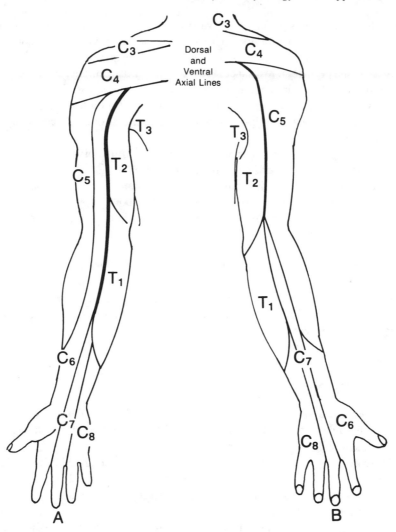

FIGURE 1-5.   Nerve root distribution of upper limb. A, on the front; B, on the back.

Maintaining adequate blood pressure in the aorta will depend on the product of two factors: peripheral resistance and cardiac output.

Resistance in the systemic circulation lies mainly in the arteries, and since resistance is based on a fourth power law, relatively small changes in the radii of arterioles will make a large difference in resistance. The smooth muscle in the arteriolar wall is in a state of partial contraction due to the continuous sympathetic nerve activity, called sympathetic or vasoconstrictor tone. This tone originates in the vasomotor center of the medulla. An increase in activity on the part of the vasomotor center will cause vasoconstriction of the peripheral vessels and an increase in the peripheral resistance. Provided the cardiac output remains constant, this will lead to a rise in blood pressure. Conversely, a decrease in the vasomotor center activity will cause a relaxation of the vasoconstrictor tone and an increase in size of the peripheral vessels—vasodilatation. If cardiac output is constant, blood pressure will fall.

Peripheral resistance depends not only on the size of the blood vessels, but also on the viscosity of the blood. It is directly proportional.

Arterial blood pressure is maintained at a constant level by the baroreceptor mechanism. Receptors in the arterial wall, which respond to pressure in the lumen of the vessel, are found in the aortic arch, in the common carotid arteries, and at the bifurcation of each of the common carotid arteries into the internal and external carotid arteries. Such receptors are termed baroreceptors. As the pressure rises, nerve impulse activity passing from these areas to the medulla increases. If the pressure falls, the impulse activity decreases. Nerve impulses run in the vagus nerve and the glossopharyngeal nerve. Other factors influencing vasomotor center activity include carbon dioxide, oxygen lack, activity of the respiratory center, tissue metabolites, and autonomic nerve system activity.

AUTONOMIC SYSTEM

The autonomic system is responsible for the innervation of glands and unstriped muscle throughout the body. It is subdivided into two functionally antagonistic systems: sympathetic and parasympathetic.

Sympathetic activity is always widespread and is characterized by an increased secretion of catecholamines, noradrenaline, and adrenalin, which act on two types of receptors in the tissues. These have been designated alpha and beta receptors. The alpha receptors are associated with the stimulation (contraction) of unstriped muscle. They are found, for example, at the termination of the postganglionic fibers to the arterioles. The beta receptors are associated with the inhibition (relaxation) of such muscle. They are also the receptors that bring about an increase in the force of contraction and rate of the heart.

The *parasympathetic* nervous system produces a local rather than a general manifestation and aims at conserving and restoring energy.

In summary, the sympathetic system is active in times of stress (id est, the "fight or flight" reaction). The parasympathetic system is more discreet and widely differing activities may be occurring simultaneously in different parts of the body. Its activity speeds up the passage of food along the digestive tract, defecation, and micturition.

HEAT AND COLD

The skin is the only organ of the body whose blood supply is not regulated according to its metabolic need. The blood flow to the skin is regulated by the heat-regulating center in the hypothalamus in the interest of body temperature regulation. Local heat produces vasodilatation by direct action on the blood vessel, and reflex dilatation may also occur in the other limb.

The effect of cold is more complex. In general it causes vasoconstriction. Constriction of the arterioles results in blood being trapped in the capillaries of the skin. This blood will lose oxygen, and the skin will become blue in color giving rise to local cyanosis. If the venous capillaries are also constricted, the skin will become white in color. Reactive hyperemia is usual following cold exposure.

NERVES

Two types of nerve fiber exist: myelinated and nonmyelinated. In the myelinated nerve fiber, the central axon is surrounded by both myelin sheath and outer neurilemma. In the nonmyelinated nerve the myelin sheath is absent and the neurilemmal sheath is the only covering to the axon. In both cases a cell nucleus termed Schwann lies under the neurilemma. In the myelinated nerves the Schwann cell has rotated many times around the axon to form the lipid protein myelin sheath. In the nonmyelinated nerve, the Schwann cell merely encloses the axon. Most of the nerves are myelinated but postganglionic autonomic fibers and other small fibers of less than 1 μg in diameter are nonmedullated.

Nerve fibers vary considerably in size and conduction velocity (Table 1-1). Nerve fibers are divided into three groups. Group A fibers are the myelinated fibers found in sensory and motor nerves. This group is further subdivided into alpha, beta, gamma, and delta on the basis of nerve fiber diameter. The large A-alpha fibers have a diameter of 15–20μ, A-beta 10–15μ and the diameter of the A-delta is as small as 2–5μ.

Group B fibers are the the preganglionic autonomic fibers, while Group C are the nonmyelinated. The latter are small, less than 2μ.

A-alpha fibers are the most easily stimulated and the velocity of conduction of myelinated fibers is proportional to the fiber diameter. A myelinated fiber conduction rate in meters per second is approximately six times the fiber diameter in microns in fibers larger than 3μ. The largest myelinated fibers with a diameter of 20μ conduct at 120 meters per second.

The nonmyelinated fibers have a conduction velocity proportional to the square root of the fiber diameter. With a diameter of 1μ, the conduction velocities are approximately the same. Below 1μ, nonmyelinated fibers have a faster conduction rate than myelinated fibers.

TABLE 1-1

| Nerve Fiber | | Velocity | Sensation |
Size	Type		
* A α15–20u	Myelinated	120 m/sec	(Motor)
β10–15u			Touch & warmth
γ5–10u			Touch
δ2–5u		3 m/sec	Sharp pain & cold
B <3u	Myelinated (pre-ganglionic autonomic)	4 m/sec	—
C 0.4–1.2u	Non-myelinated (Postganglionic autonomic and some terminal)	1–3 m/sec	Burning pain & warmth

Key: * most easily stimulated.

During the spike potential, the nerve fiber is absolutely refractory, and no stimulus, no matter how strong, can initiate a fresh impulse. The nerve is inexcitable. This is followed by a partial refractory state when only a very strong stimulus can excite, and this produces a subnormal spike. Large fibers recover in 1 millisecond and therefore could theoretically propagate 1,000 impulses per second.

The refractory state is followed by the negative after-potential state, during which the nerve is hyperexcitable. This is followed by the positive after-potential state, during which time the nerve is in a subnormal state of excitability.

When a nerve reaches striated muscle fiber, it loses its myelin sheath and the bare axon ramifies with the muscle sarcoplasm forming a motor end-plate.

If the contracting muscle is allowed to shorten under a steady load, the contraction is termed isotonic. Contraction without shortening is termed isometric. Voluntary movements are a mixture of both (for example, lifting a heavy weight is mainly isotonic contraction, but holding it in mid-air involves an isometric contraction of the muscles).

PERIPHERAL SENSIBILITY OF THE HAND

The sensory ending of a nerve may be a "free" ending, a nerve network, or an ending in relationship to a nonneural structure. These nonneural structures may be hairy follicles or a form of "encapsulated end organ." The encapsulated end organs are Pacinian or Meissner corpuscles, and Merkel cell-neurite complexes. The distribution in human skin is seen in Figure 1-6.

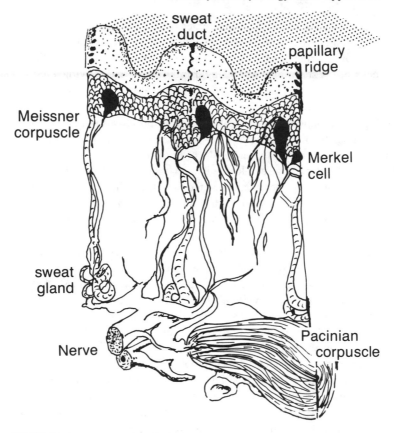

FIGURE 1-6.   Cross section of skin illustrating site of mechanoreceptors.

The *Pacinian corpuscle* is a deep dermal and subcutaneous sensory receptor 1-4 mm long and 0.5-1 mm wide innervated by a single myelinated nerve. Estimates of the number of corpuscles present vary from 200 per thumb, 600 per hand, 120 per cm of volar pulp. The axon enters the corpuscle, loses its myelin sheath and enters the inner core. The axon is surrounded by 40-60 concentric lamellae. The Pacinian corpuscle may occasionally be bilobed. This is the receptor for 2-point discrimination and vibration above 60 Hz. It is insensitive to thermal stimuli.

The *Meissner corpuscle* is an encapsulated, oval end organ within the dermal papillary ridge and more specifically the intermediary ridge. They may be bilobed but most commonly a single-lobed corpuscle is present. Within each lobulation, there appears to be a stacked series of flattened discs, which in effect represent the lamellar cells. The nuclei usually appear at the edge or side of the capsule. Each corpuscle is innervated by two to nine separate nerve fibers. Two to three fibers enter at the base, and the others enter from its sides or top. The fibers lose their myelin sheaths as they enter the corpuscle, and the lamellar cells may represent either perineural (Schwann) cells or modified epithelial cells or both. These cells are best stimulated by fingertip stroking and moving 2-point esthesiometry. They are the receptors for thermal sensation and low-frequency vibration (below 60 Hz).

Multiple fiber innovation of the Meissner corpuscle allows for overlap of the peripheral receptor fields of individual fibers in a manner not possible with the Pacinian corpuscle or the Merkel cell-Neurite complex.

The *Merkel cell* is a large cell located in the basal layer of the epidermis. In hairy skin it is either in groups below an elevated pad (haarscheibe) or associated with a hair (tylotrich or vibrissae), while in the glabrous (nonhairy) digital skin it lies in groups of four in the basal layer about the entrance of the sweat duct into the intermediate ridge. A single myelinated nerve innovates a haarscheibe in humans, and a group of Merkel cells about the sweat duct in the glabrous skin. Although it had been suggested at one time that the Pacinian corpuscle was the pressure receptor, only a slowly adapting fiber/receptor system such as the Merkel cell-neurite complex is responsive to vertical skin displacement in a linear fashion. These cells best detect classic 2-point discrimination, and fingertip touch and pressure.

The number of nerve fibers present in a given area of skin is referred to as the peripheral innervation density and is related to the volume of cerebral cortex representing that area. Thus, for example, the hand, and in particular the fingertips, have among the highest innervation density of any place on the body surface and are represented by one of the largest areas on the sensory cortex. In the peripheral nerve the A-alpha are motor fibers, the A-beta fibers are correlated with touch, the A-delta with pricking pain and temperature, and the C fibers with burning pain.

The A-beta fibers can be subdivided based on their adaptation to a constant-touch stimulus (Table 1-2). A fiber is termed rapidly adapting if its impulse response drops off rapidly to zero. A fiber is termed slowly adapting if its pulse response continues throughout the stimulus duration. Only the slowly adapting fibers increase their rate of firing, or impulse frequency, as the stimulus intensity is increased. Thus only a slowly adapting fiber can convey information regarding constant touch and pressure, and the receptors are the Merkel cell-neutrite. They are stimulated by direct pressure or deflection of an associated hair. The Weber test, classical 2-point discrimination, in which the blunt ends of a caliper are held in constant contact with the skin, measures the innervation density of the slowly adapting fiber/receptor population. The quickly adapting fiber conveys information about movement. Thus, the quickly adapting fiber/receptor system detects moving touch. The "moving 2-point discrimination test," in which the two ends of the caliper are moved, measures the peripheral innervation density of the quickly adapting fiber/receptor system.

TABLE 1-2

Sensory Nerve Fibre Size and Property	Mechanoreceptor	Site	Innervation	Sensation	Clincial Test
A-Beta Slow-adapting (SA 1 & 2)	Merkel cell-neurite complex	Basal layer of epidermis	Single nerve	Constant touch and pressure Tactile sharp edge Tactile gap 1mm	Finger touch Depth sense 2-point discrimination
A-Beta Fast adapting (FA 1)	Meissner corpuscle	Dermal papillary ridge	Multiple	Moving touch Vibration 5-60Hz Tactile sharp edge Tactile gap <5mm	Finger tip stroking Tuning fork 30cps Vibrometer Depth sense 2 point discrimination Neurometer CTP 5Hz
A-Beta Fast-adapting (FA 11)	Pacinian corpuscle	Deep dermal and substaneous	Single nerve	Moving touch Vibration 60-400 Hz Tactile sharp edge Tactile gap >5mm	Finger tip stroking Tuning fork 256cps Vibrometer Depth sense 2 point discrimination Neurometer CTP 250 Hz

The mechanoreceptor, an end organ, is actually a transducer. It transforms a mechanical stimulus into a conducted neural impulse. While the exact mechanism of this transducer process remains to be defined, the mechanoreceptors signal to the sensory cortex by a frequency code (that is, a temporal pattern of impulses). The slowly adapting fiber/receptor systems have two neurophysiological properties. The first is that the neural impulses continue to discharge throughout the duration of the stimulus, although the frequency diminishes with duration. The second is that there is a change in response (frequency of impulse) with stimulus intensity change. Thus when the mechanical probe is pushed deeper into the skin there are more frequent neural discharges recorded from the so-called type 1 slowly adapting receptors. The slow-adaptors are the pressure sensors.

A type 2 fiber/receptor system that responds to lateral displacement from stretching of skin adjacent to its receptive field is uncommon. In addition to responding to constant touch and pressure, slowly adapting receptors may respond to changes in temperature, but they do not convey the perception of temperature. At the level of the digital nerve, there are 2,500 axons, and it has been estimated that about 10 percent to 36 percent of A-betas are slowly adapting.

The quickly adapting fiber/receptor systems are related to Pacinian and Meissner corpuscles, and although the Pacinian corpuscle is insensitive to thermal stimulation, it has rapid properties of adaptation. If a vibratory stimulus (an oscillating mechanical probe, electrical sine wave, or tuning fork) is applied to the peripheral receptive field of a quickly adapting fiber, a threshold (amplitude wave) will be found for that frequency at which the stimulus is transmitted. This is the absolute threshold at which an action potential is generated.

Another phenomenon is flutter-vibration. The quickly adapting population of group A-beta fibers in glabrous skin contains one group more sensitive to low-frequency stimuli (range of 5 to 40 cps), maximally sensitive to about 30 cps, and another group most sensitive to high-frequency stimuli (range of 60 to 300 cps), maximally sensitive to about 250 cps. From studies it has been concluded that one subset of the quickly adapting fibers responsive to low-frequency stimuli have their receptors located in the epidermis (probably the Meissner corpuscle). They are also responsible for detecting transient stimuli (movement) and flutter. The second subset of quickly adapting fibers responsive to high-frequency stimuli have their receptors located below the epidermis (probably the Pacinian corpuscles), and they are responsible for detecting transients (movement) and vibration. Pacinian corpuscles are more sensitive than Meissner corpuscles and have a larger receptive field. In glaborous skin they may only constitute 6 percent of the receptors. Pacinian afferents are not present in hairy skin. Thus cutaneous sensibility is organized according to specific fiber/receptor systems. There is evidence suggesting that the specific profile of neural impulses generated at the fingertip reach the thalamic level essentially unchanged.

SUMMARY

The anatomy of blood vessels and nerves of the upper limb is described, with particular emphasis on the hands where HAV-exposure will have most effect. The types of nerve fibers (A, B, and C) and the mechanoreceptors (Pacinian, Meissner, and Merkel) for peripheral sensitivity are described, and their function discussed.

The factors that influence blood circulation in the peripheral arteries include blood carbon dioxide, oxygen, and metabolites; activity of the respiratory and vasomotor centers in the brain stem; and sensory impulses, particularly pain.

The autonomic system is subdivided into two functionally antagonistic systems: sympathetic and parasympathetic. The sympathetic outflow is limited to the thoracic and upper lumbar segments of the spinal cord from T_1 to L_2. Sympathetic activity is always widespread and noradrenaline and adrenaline is released to act on alpha and beta receptors in the tissues. Nerve fibers are of three types. Groups A and B are myelinated, and C are nonmyelinated. Their combined function is responsible for touch, pain, and hot and cold sensation. The nerves end in mechanoreceptors consisting of Merkel cell-neurite complex (slowly adapting), Meissner corpuscles, and Pacinian corpuscles (both fast adapting). The neurophysiological response from these receptors differ, and are identified by their sensory responses.

Bibliography

Warwick, R. *Johnston's Synopsis of Regional Anatomy.* 9th ed. Philadelphia: Lea & Febiger, 1963:449.

Green, J. H. *An Introduction to Human Physiology.* 4th ed. London: Oxford University Press, 1977:232.

Doscher, W.; Viswanathan, B.; Stein, T.; Margolis, I. B. "Hemodynamic Assessment of the Circulation of 200 Normal Hands." *Ann. Surg.* 1983; 198:776-779.

Coffman, J. D. "Total and Nutritional Blood Flow in the Finger." *Clin. Sci.* 1972; 42:243-250.

Mountcastle, V. B.; LaMotte, R. H.; Carli, G. "Detection Thresholds for Stimuli in Humans and Monkeys: Comparison With Threshold Events in Mechanoreceptive Afferent Nerve Fibres Innervating the Monkey Hand." *J. Neurophysiol.* 1972; 35:122-136.

Mountcastle, V. B. "The View From Within: Pathways to the Study of Perception." *Johns Hopkins Med. J.* 1975; 136:109-131.

Mountcastle, V. B. "Sensory Receptors and Neural Encodings: Introduction to Sensory Processes." In: Mountcastle, V. B., ed. *Medical Physiology.* 14th ed. St. Louis: CV Mosby, 1980; 1(v):327-347.

Mountcastle, V. B. "Neural Mechanisms in Somesthesis." In: Mountcastle, V. B., ed. *Medical Physiology.* 14th ed. St. Louis: CV Mosby, 1980; 1(v):348-390.

Mountcastle, V. B. "Pain and Temperature Sensibilities." In: Mountcastle, V. B., ed. *Medical Physiology.* 14th ed. St. Louis: CV Mosby, 1980; 1(v):391-427.

Lundstrom, R. J. I. "Responses of Mechanoreceptive Afferent Units in the Glabrous Skin of the Human Hand to Vibration." *Scand. J. Work. Environ. Health* 1986; 12:413-416.

2

Raynaud's Phenomenon

P. L. Pelmear

Raynaud's phenomenon, named after Maurice Raynaud (1834–1881), may be defined as intermittent constriction of the peripheral vessels—arterioles and veins—with consequent color change of the skin of the extremities, pallor, cyanosis or both. This phenomenon, commonly precipitated by exposure to cold, may occur primarily as in Raynaud's disease, or in association with a number of conditions or diseases.

PRIMARY RAYNAUD'S DISEASE

Maurice Raynaud received his doctorate degree from the Faculty of Medicine in Paris in 1862 for a thesis entitled "De L' Asphyxie Locale et de la Gangréne Symetrique Des Extremites." In the thesis he described very clearly the episodes of discoloration of the digits and his name has been associated with the phenomenon ever since. In 1874, he published further research on the subject, and both the latter and the thesis have been translated into English.[1] Raynaud attempted to demonstrate that there existed a variety of dry gangrene affecting the extremities that was impossible to explain by a vascular obstruction—a variety characterized especially by a remarkable tendency to symmetry. For many years, "Raynaud's disease" was used as a convenient label for cases of obscure etiology in which intermittent pallor, cyanosis, pain, or gangrene of the hands, feet, nose, or ears were symptoms. Although Raynaud defined his symptoms clearly enough, he included many cases in his thesis and subsequent report that were not representative (for example, patients with leukemia, tuberculosis, diabetes, arteriosclerosis, hemiplegia and sclerodactyly).[2] Subsequently, it was appreciated that although Raynaud's disease was a clinical entity, the blanching of digits (that is Raynaud's phenomenon) is commonly associated with many different conditions. Hence we recognize

18

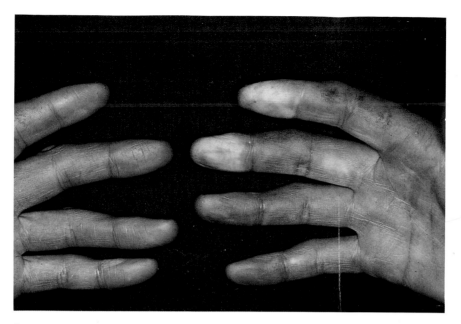

Stage 1 Blanching of finger tips.

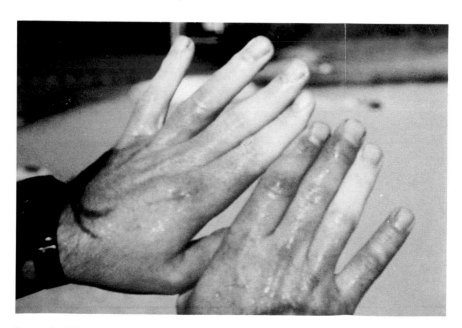

Stage 2 Blanching to base of middle phalanx.

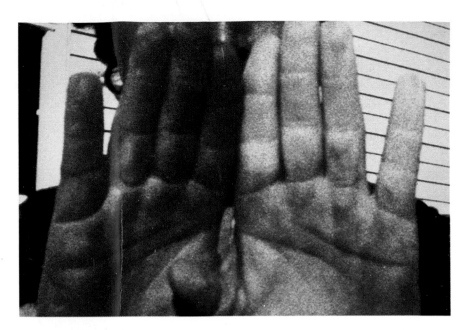

Stage 3 Blanching to base of fingers.

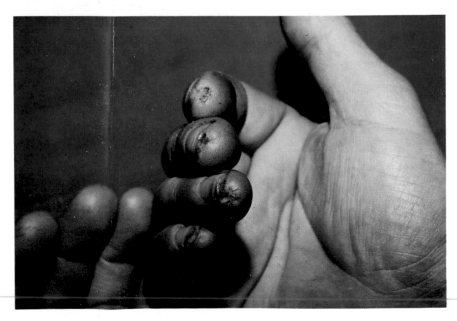

Stage 4 Trophic lesion of finger tip.

Raynaud's phenomenon in the former as primary, and with the other conditions as secondary.

The distinguishing features of Raynaud's disease are now well defined.[3] The age of onset is usually 11 to 45 years and 77 percent are female. The blanching of the fingers is usually bilateral and cyanosis may be seen before or after the blanching, followed by redness when recovering from the attack. Blanching when fully established normally extends to the base of all fingers and may even involve the tips of the thumbs and palms of the hands. In 50-61 percent of cases, fingers only are affected; in 36–43 percent toes and fingers. The nose, ears, face, chest and lips are reported to be affected in some patients.[4] Cold exposure is the commonest cause of the vasospastic attacks, but emotional stress may be an additional precipitating cause in up to 60 percent. In addition, pressure on the fingers, together with cold exposure, is one of the most common instigating factors. About 13 percent of patients have trophic changes of the digits.[5]

The prevalence of Raynaud's disease in the community will depend on the climatic conditions in different temperature zones, and it may be as high as 30 percent but is usually at least 10 percent in temperate zones. The disease in men is similar to that in women, although fewer men are affected, and male subjects in industry usually have a prevalence of 5–6 percent.

Prognosis is dependent on a number of factors. Movement to a warmer climate will eliminate symptoms in the majority, and although tobacco smoking is better avoided it does not seem to affect the prognosis. Treatment with sympatholytic agents and calcium-blocking drugs have yielded the best results, with improvement occurring in about 50 percent of patients. It has been reported that using two drugs that act by different mechanisms to produce vasodilation yields more benefit than one agent.[6] Cervical sympathectomy used to be a popular surgical procedure, but sympathectomy should only be considered now for lower limb vasospastic disease.

The diagnosis of Raynaud's disease normally has to be made from a careful history as it is difficult to produce blanching of the skin in the office or the laboratory. Vascular tests (see Chapter 5) are able to demonstrate vasospasm, but such tests are not normally justified for minor cases of Raynaud's disease. The physical examination is usually normal in such patients although the hands or feet may be cool. Because vasospastic attacks may precede diagnostic criteria of connective tissue diseases by several years, particularly scleroderma, clinicians have relied on the criteria proposed by Allen and Brown[7] for the diagnosis of Raynaud's disease.

1. Onset in the younger age group, that is, under 30 years.
2. Vasospastic attacks precipitated by exposure to cold or emotional stimuli.
3. Bilateral involvement of the extremities.
4. Absence of gangrene or, if present, limited to the skin of fingertips.

5. No evidence of an underlying disease that could be responsible for vasospastic attacks.
6. History of symptoms for at least two years.

Fewer patients with connective tissue disease are missed if criterion 5 includes normal levels of antinuclear antibodies, erythrocyte sedimentation rate (ESR), nail fold capillaroscopy, pulmonary function, and esophageal motility studies. This work up can be expensive, and probably should be reserved for patients presenting with severe vasospastic attacks, ulcers, or gangrene, and men and women who first develop the syndrome after age 40.[8] In the community, Raynaud's disease accounts for most cases of Raynaud's phenomenon, as evidenced by the small incidence of connective tissue disease and other secondary causes.[9]

Pathophysiology of Raynaud's Disease

Raynaud's disease may occur in several members of a family, suggesting a hereditary or genetic factor. Raynaud concluded that there was no obstacle to the flow of the blood inside the capillaries but that the circulation was "slackened," and that the symptoms were caused by a spasm of the capillary vessels, due to overactivity of the sympathetic nervous system. This theory of sympathetic hyperactivity was challenged in 1929 by Lewis[10] who proposed that there was a "local fault" within the digital arteries themselves. He considered that intimal thicking and thrombosis of digital vessels contributed to the diminished blood flow. Following thrombotic or embolic processes, a blood vessel may fail to become fully patent and subsequent normal increases of tone, such as are induced by cold, will cause transient or conspicuous reduction of blood flow. He postulated that the original disturbance may be a sudden and nonrecurring event, leaving behind it a proneness to attacks of cyanosis, which wrongly came to be regarded as signifying active disease. Additional evidence in support of the local theory is that reflex sympathetic vasoconstriction is enhanced in patients with primary Raynaud's disease by locally cooling the hand, but not in normal subjects.[11] The authors considered that the most likely explanation for the greater decrease in blood flow of the cooled hand in patients with Raynaud's disease was that cold temperatures sensitized the alpha-adrenoreceptor-mediated vasoconstriction of vascular smooth muscle. Thermal-entrainment studies have also supported a local fault in that Raynaud's disease patients have abnormal vascular responses in one hand when the contralateral hand is alternatively warmed and cooled at low frequencies.[12] Hyperviscosity as a factor in Raynaud's disease has been suggested.[13]

Vasospasm ensues when vessel wall tone overcomes the intraluminal pressure. Any proximal obstruction that reduces this pressure is therefore likely to be associated with distal vasospasm. In the primary disease, structural abnormalities have not been demonstrated in the digital vessels, so the local sensitivity of the digital arteries to cold seems to indicate that the abnormality may lie in the alpha-adrenoreceptors.

The other distinctive feature of Raynaud's disease is the prolonged vasospasm that occurs. Lafferty and co-workers[14] have shown that local temperature changes produce distant effects in the blood flow of the opposite hand, which are mediated by the hypothalamus through the sympathetic nervous system (that is, thermal entrainment). In thermal-entrainment studies the blood flow traces obtained indicate that whereas in normal subjects the blood vessels constrict and rapidly vasodilate after each thermally induced sympathetic response, in Raynaud's patients this rapid "postsympathetic" vasodilation is delayed or absent. Vasodilation occurs only when a warm stimulus is applied. They suggest that there are two systems, one producing a coarse and the other a fine control of blood flow. An increase in sympathetic tone arising from the hypothalamus (coarse control) causes vasoconstriction through alpha-adrenergic stimulation of the alpha-1 and alpha-2 receptors in the blood vessels, but it also affects the mast-cell membrane producing a release of histamine and vasodilation (fine control) after a delay of seconds. The sympathetic nerve terminal in the arterioles have histamine H_2 receptors, which inhibit alpha-adrenergic transmission. They therefore suggest that with Raynaud's disease the "local fault" is in the histaminergic vasodilating system. The overall decrease in available tissue histamine will permit the prolonged vasospasm.[15] The relative contributions of autonomic, humoral, and local mechanisms in the pathophysiology of Raynaud's disease remain unknown. Such a variable list of disease associated with the same physical signs and symptoms of intermittent digital vasospasm (that is, Raynaud's phenomenon) suggests a common final pathway of vasomotor disturbance.

SECONDARY CAUSES OF RAYNAUD'S PHENOMENON

Trauma

Hand-Arm vibration Syndrome   (HAVS) (see chapters 3, 4, 5, 6) resulting from HAV exposure is the most common cause. However, any trauma to the digital vessels leading to section, occlusion, or thrombosis (for example, following frostbite, may subsequently cause a reduction of finger systolic pressure with subsequent Raynaud's phenomenon on cold exposure.

Similarly, compression of the proximal blood vessels may have the same effect when it occurs as a result of *cervical ribs or thoracic outlet syndrome.*[16] In most of the latter cases the neurological symptoms predominate because of compression of the brachial plexus.[17] To confirm the diagnosis, extensive noninvasive vascular and neurological tests are essential.[18, 19] Surgery is rarely indicated in thoracic outlet syndrome[20] but is beneficial for a cervical rib.

Intoxication

Drugs   that block the beta-adrenoreceptors are the most common agents that induce Raynaud's phenomenon. Such drugs are used for treating hypertensive patients and the incidence of Raynaud's phenomenon or cold extremities may be as high as 40 percent.[21, 22] Such patients should be provided with alternative therapy.

Ergot and ergotamine preparations have long been known to produce intense vasospasm by stimulating the alpha-adrenoreceptors to which the drug is tightly bound.[23] It is usually associated with excessive doses of the drug. Bleomycin, and Vinblastine therapy for testicular carcinomas, lymphomas, and head or neck tumors may produce Raynaud's phenomenon in up to 37 percent of patients.[24]

Workers who were involved in the production of *vinyl chloride*, particularly those who had to clean the vats, developed a multisystem disease resembling scleroderma. The predominant symptom was Reynaud's phenomenon with acro-osteolysis, but excessive fatigue, aches in bones, joints and muscles, dyspnea and loss of libido were other common symptoms.[25] Removal from exposure resulted in partial recovery and recalcification of the phalangeal bones.[26]

Obstructive Arterial Disease

Patients with degenerative vascular disease affecting the peripheral circulation, often in conjunction with diabetes, may have associated Raynaud's phenomenon.

Connective Tissue Diseases

Any of the connective tissue diseases that affect skin, joints, and internal organs may be associated with Raynaud's phenomenon. Of these, rheumatoid arthritis and systemic sclerosis are the most important.

Rheumatoid Arthritis
In this disease mottled discoloration and cool sweaty hands on exposure to cold is more common than classical Raynaud's phenomenon. Dry eyes and mouth, and enlargement of salivary or lacrimal glands suggest Sjögren's syndrome. Secondary *Sjögren's syndrome* may occur in association with several diseases but most frequently with rheumatoid arthritis and systemic lupus erythematosus. These patients may test positive for rheumatoid factor and have elevated antinuclear antibody, with antibodies to nucleoprotein antigens SS-B and SS-A.

Systemic Sclerosis
The epidemiological study of this condition has been hampered by its relative rarity (less than 12 per million), considerable clinical variability, difficulty in diagnosis, and frequency with which its features overlap with other clinically related disorders

such as systemic erythematosus and polymyositis-dermatomyositis. Systemic sclerosis represents a broad spectrum of disease ranging from widespread severe skin thickening (diffuse scleroderma), skin thickening limited to the distal extremities and face (limited scleroderma), or absent skin thickening (systemic sclerosis sine scleroderma).[27] Vasospastic attacks typical of Raynaud's phenomenon or persistent vasospasm manifested by cyanosis during cold exposure occurs in 90 percent of patients with scleroderma or systemic sclerosis.[28] It is the presenting symptom in almost 50 percent of patients. Digital tip ulceration or gangrene is a severe complication. While systemic sclerosis is rare in children and in men under age 30, the incidence increases steadily with age, peaking between ages 45 and 64.[29] Most studies show a two-to-three-fold excess of systemic sclerosis in women. A familial association is suggested by reports of systemic sclerosis occurring in first degree relatives like other autoimmune diseases such as rheumatoid arthritis and systemic lupus erythematosus.[30]

Secondary causes of Raynaud's phenomenon are as follows:

1. *Trauma*
    a. Direct to extremities
       HAVS
       Lacerations with blood vessel injury
       Frostbite and immersion syndrome
    b. Compression of proximal blood vessels
       Thoracic outlet syndrome
       Cervical rib
       Costoclavicular and hyperabduction syndrome
2. *Intoxication*
    a. Drug Therapy
       Beta-adrenoreceptor blocking agents
       Ergot preparations
       Methysergide
       Bleomycin and Vinblastine
    b. Vinyl chloride (acro-osteolysis)
3. *Obstructive Arterial Disease*
    a. Arteriosclerosis obliterans
    b. Thromboangitis obliterans
    c. Arterial emboli
4. *Connective Tissue Diseases*
    a. Rheumatoid arthritis and Sjögren's syndrome
    b. Scleroderma (cutaneous-limited and diffuse; CREST)
    c. Systemic lupus erythematosus
    d. Mixed connective tissue disease
    e. Polymyositis and dermatomyositis

5. *Hypersensitivity*
   a. Cryoglobulinemia
   b. Cold agglutinins
   c. Cryofibrinogenemia
   d. Paraproteinaemia

SUMMARY

Raynaud's phenomenon or blanching of the digits is commonly precipitated by exposure to cold, and it may occur primarily as in Raynaud's disease, or in association with a number of conditions or diseases. Raynaud's Disease, which is more common in women than men, is familial, and the prevalence in the community is at least 10 percent.

The most common secondary cause is HAVS, which develops following exposure to vibrating tools. Local trauma to the digital vessels or compression of the proximal blood vessels by cervical ribs or musculature, as in the thoracic outlet syndrome, are common causes.

Drug therapy with beta-blockers, ergot preparations, Bleomycin, and Vinblastine is sometimes associated with Raynaud's phenomenon, and vinyl chloride intoxication has also been a cause. Raynaud's phenomenon may occur with peripheral arterial disease, and is commonly a presenting symptom with the collagen diseases, particularly systemic sclerosis and rheumatoid arthritis.

Notes

1. Raynaud, M. "Local Asphyxia and Symmetrical gangrene of the extremities" (MD Thesis). Paris, 1862. Translated into English by the New Sydenham Society and published in selective Monographs. London 1888.
2. Hunt, J. H. "The Raynaud's Phenomena: A Critical Review." *Quart. J. Med. New Series.* 1936; 19(5):399–444.
3. Coffman, J. D. *Raynaud's Phenomenon.* London: Oxford University Press, 1989:186.
4. Grifford, R. W., Jr. and Hines, E. A., Jr. "Raynaud's Disease Among Women and Girls." *Circulation* 1957; 16(2):1012–1021.
5. Ibid
6. Coffman, *Raynaud's Phenomenon.*
7. Allen, E. V.; Brown, G. E. "Raynaud's Disease: A Critical Review of Minimal Requisites for Diagnosis." *Am. J. Med. Sci.* 1932; 183:187–200.
8. Coffman, J. D. "Evaluation of a Patient with Raynaud's Phenomenon." *Postgrad. Med.* 1985; 78(2):175–183.
9. Silman, A.; Holligan, S.; Brennan, P.; Maddison, P. "Prevalence of Symptoms of Raynaud's Phenomenon in General Practice." *BMJ* 1990; 301:590–592.
10. Lewis, T. "Experiments Related to the Peripheral Mechanisms Involved in the Spastic Arrest of the Circulation in the Fingers of Raynaud's Disease." *Heart* 1929; 15:7–100.

11. Jamieson, G. G.; Ludbrook, J.; Wilson, A. "Cold Hypersensitivity in Raynaud's Phenomenon." *Circulation* 1971; 44(2):254-264.

12. Lafferty, K.; De Trafford, J. C.; Roberts, V. C.; Cotton, L. T. "Raynaud's Phenomenon and Thermal Entrainment: An Objective Test." *BMJ* 1983; 286:90-92.

13. Pringle, R.; Walder, D. N.; Weaver, J. P. A. "Blood Viscosity and Raynaud's disease." *Lancet* 1965; 1:1086-1089.

14. Lafferty, K.; De Trafford, J. C.; Roberts, V. C.; and Cotton, L. T.; "Raynaud's Phenomenon."

15. Lafferty, K.; De Trafford, J. C.; Roberts, V. C.; Cotton, L. T. "On the Nature of Raynaud's Phenomenon: The Role of Histamine." *Lancet* 1983; 2:313-315.

16. Ruckley, C.V. "Thoracic Outlet Syndrome." *BMJ* 1983; 287:447-448.

17. Gilliatt, R. W. "Thoracic Outlet Syndrome." *BMJ* 1983; 287:764.

18. Rush, M. P.; McNally, D. M.; Rossmann, M. E.; Otis, S. "Non-invasive Vascular Diagnosis of Thoracic Outlet Syndrome." *Bruit* 1983; 7:56-59.

19. Veilleux, M.; Stevens, J. C.; Campbell, J. K. "Somatosensory Evoked Potentials: Lack of Value for Diagnosis of Thoracic Outlet Syndrome." *Muscle Nerve* 1988; 11(6):571-575.

20. Cherington, M. "Surgery for Thoracic Outlet Syndrome?" *New Eng. J. Med.* 1986; 314(5):322.

21. Feleke, E.; Lyngstam, O.; Rastam, L.; Ryden, L. "Complaints of Cold Extremities Among Patients on Antihypertensive Treatment." *Acta. Med. Scand.* 1983; 213(5):381-385.

22. Marshall, A. J.; Roberts, C. J. C.; Barritt, D. W. "Raynaud's Phenomenon as Side Effect of Beta-Blockers in Hypertension." *BMJ* 1976; 1:1498-1499.

23. Innes, I. R. "Identification of the Smooth Muscle Excitatory Receptors for Ergot Alkaloids." *Brit. J. Pharmacol.* 1962; 19:120-128.

24. Vogelzang, N. J.; Bosl, G. J.; Johnson, K.; Kennedy, B. J. "Raynaud's Phenomenon: A Common Toxicity After Combination Chemotherapy for Testicular Cancer." *Ann. Intern. Med.* 1981; 95(3):288-292.

25. Vale, P. T.; Kipling, M. D.; Walker, A. "Miscellaneous Symptoms Occurring in Workers Engaged in the Manufacturer of PVC." *J. Soc. Occup. Med.* 1976; 26:95-97.

26. Stewart, J. D.; Williams, D. M. J.; McLachlan, M. S. F. "Acro-Osteolysis in a Polyvinyl Chloride Worker With an Atypical Industrial History." *J. Soc. Occup. Med.* 1975; 25:103-109.

27. Steen, V. D.; Medsger, T. A. "Epidemiology and Natural History of Systemic Sclerosis." In: LeRoy, E. C., ed. *Rheumatic Disease Clinics of North America.* Philadelphia: WB Saunders, 1990; 16(1):1-10.

28. Tuffanelli, D. L.; and Winkelmann, R. K. "Systemic Scleroderma: A Clinical Study of 727 Cases." *Arch. Dermatol.* 1961; 84:359-371.

29. Medsger, T. A., Jr.; and Masi, A. T. "Epidemiology of Systemic Sclerosis (Scleroderma). *Ann. Intern. Med.* 1971; 74(5):714-721.

30. Flores, R. H.; Stevens, M. B.; Arnett, F. C. "Familial Occurrence of Progressive Systemic Sclerosis and Systemic Lupus Erythematosus." *J. Rheumatol.* 1984; 11(3):321-323.

3

Clinical Picture (Vascular, Neurological, and Musculoskeletal)

P. L. Pelmear, W. Taylor

HAND-ARM VIBRATION SYNDROME

Hand-arm vibration syndrome (HAVS) is a new term for a condition known since the early 1900s. The following terms have been used: traumatic vasospastic disease, dead man's hand, spastic anemia, Raynaud's phenomenon of occupational origin, and vibration induced white finger (VWF). Hand-arm vibration syndrome was defined in 1983 by scientists at an international meeting in London, England,[1] as a disease entity with the following peripheral components:

Circulatory disturbances (vasospasm with local finger blanching "white finger"),
Sensory and Motor disturbances (numbness, loss of finger coordination and dexterity, clumsiness and inability to perform intricate tasks.), and
Musculo-skeletal disturbances (muscle, bone and joint disorders).

Vibration as a cause of Raynaud's phenomenon was first reported by Loriga in 1911,[2] but the earliest full description in the literature of workers with vibration-induced Raynaud's phenomenon is by Dr. Alice Hamilton.[3] She examined 181 stonecutters and carvers at the limestone quarries in Bedford, Indiana, United States, and her noteworthy description of the injuries to the hands has stood the test of time, and she is unsurpassed for her clinical descriptions.

Symptoms and Signs

Vascular Effects
After a variable period of time, depending on the intensity of the vibration received, the vibration exposure time and the susceptibility of the subject, blanching of a fingertip occurs following exposure to cold. With increasing vibration dosage, the

26

blanching progresses to the bases of the fingers. The blanching attacks are usually precipitated by exposure to cold damp conditions, particularly in the morning and at night, when the subjects metabolic activity is low; following the handling of cold objects or immersion in water; and are more common in winter than in summer, but eventually they will occur all year round. With continued exposure to vibration the blanching attacks become more frequent. Typically they last for a few minutes to one hour and terminate with reactive hyperemia and often considerable pain. During an attack, the affected fingers feel numb as touch, pain, and temperature sensitivity are often greatly reduced, and in some subjects this may persist causing permanent impairment.

Initially, the blanching is localized to the tips of the fingers most exposed to the vibration source, but eventually it spreads to involve all fingers as far as the metacarpo-phalangeal joints and the tips of the thumb. The palms of the hands are rarely affected. The blanching does not usually occur at work except during rest periods, but in some subjects the vibration stimulus itself will induce blanching if the fingers are cold.

These symptoms and signs are in response to pathological and physiological changes in the tissues of the fingers. The developmental process whereby the digital vessels become sensitive to a cold stimulus is not entirely clear, and several hypotheses have been proposed (see Chapter 4).

The symptoms and signs, and the frequency of attacks may be such that the subject, apart from taking immediate preventive action to keep warm and avoid cold exposure, has to curtail his or her domestic and leisure activities. Socially this may mean avoiding outdoor pursuits such as gardening, fishing, golfing, bowling, swimming, and watching outdoor entertainment. Ultimately, it may involve a change of work to avoid further vibration exposure. Job selection in the future will be limited to warm environments.

A grading index by stage of symptoms and social/work interference was derived by Taylor and Pelmear in 1968.[4] It proved to be very useful to express clinically the stage of severity of VWF and to monitor improvement or progression in affected subjects. The Taylor-Pelmear grading did not directly address the neurological effects except in respect of the social, domestic, and leisure activities and lack of manual dexterity. The only reference was OT/ON (see Table 3-1) and this symptom grade was devised for the early vascular neuropathy. The episodes of ischemia cause a reaction of the nerve endings resulting in pain and tingling following vasospasm, and these symptoms are often complained of by subjects prior to developing HAVS, especially at night when hand circulation is sluggish (i.e., nocturnal paraesthesiae). These subjects awaken because of numbness and discomfort in their hands and fingers, and have to swing their arms and rub their fingers to improve the peripheral circulation.

Placing the subjects in stages 1 to 3 was a judgmental decision by the examiner. It was based on the number of digits affected, the extent of the blanching, the

TABLE 3-1   Stages of VWF

Stage	Condition of Digits	Work and Social Interference
0	No blanching of digits.	No complaints.
OT or ON	Intermittent tingling, numbness, or both.	No interference with activities.
I	Blanching of one or more fingertips with or without tingling and numbness.	No interference with activities.
2	Blanching of one or more fingers with numbness. Usually confined to winter.	Slight interference with home and social activities. No interference at work.
3	Extensive blanching. Frequent episodes, summer as well as winter.	Definite interference at work, at home and with social activities. Restriction of hobbies.
4	Extensive blanching. Most fingers; frequent episodes, summer and winter.	Occupation changed to avoid further vibration exposure because of severity of symptoms and signs.

frequency of blanching attacks as well as interference with home, social, and work activities, in conjunction with clinical and objective test findings. The Subjects became stage 4 when they changed occupation to avoid further exposure because of the severity of their conditions.

Although many international investigators began to use this staging, difficulties were experienced because subjects could reduce the frequency of the attacks and extent of blanching by administrative controls (for example, avoidance of cold, use of warmer clothing, gloves), and some subjects discontinued work at stage 2 to avoid further deterioration, so stage 4 by definition was inappropriate. The summer/winter differentiation did not apply to all countries. There was difficulty quantifying the subject's interference with domestic, social, and hobby activities. Furthermore there was evidence from several sources that the various pathological components of the syndrome may develop independently[5-8] so a separate classification for peripheral vascular and neurological disturbances was desirable. International researchers at a workshop in Stockholm, Sweden, in 1986 called for a revision of the Taylor-Pelmear classification and agreed to support a separate staging system for the vascular (Table 3-2)[9] and the sensorineural (Table 3-3)[10] effects.

The Stockholm vascular staging is based on the history as given by the subject. Environmental interferences are not considered. Stages 1 and 2 have occasional white finger attacks affecting one or more fingers and are distinguished by the extent of blanching. Stage 3 has frequent attacks affecting all phalanges of most fingers. Stage 4 is distinguished by the presence of trophic skin changes. The staging is made separately for each hand. In the evaluation of the subject, the grade of the disorder is indicated by the stages of both hands, and the number of affected fingers on each hand, (for example 2L(2) 1R(1)).

TABLE 3-2   The Stockholm Workshop Scale for the Classification of Cold-Induced Raynaud's Phenomenon in the Hand-Arm Vibration Syndrome.[a]

Stage	Grade	Description
0		No attacks.
1	Mild	Occasional attacks affecting only the tips of one or more fingers.
2	Moderate	Occasional attacks affecting distal and middle (rarely also proximal) phalanges of one or more fingers.
3	Severe	Frequent attacks affecting all phalanges of most fingers.
4	Very severe	As in stage 3, with trophic skin changes in the finger tips.

[a]The staging is made separately for each hand. In the evaluation of the subject, the grade of the disorder is indicated by the stages of both hands and the number of affected fingers on each hand; example: "2L(2)/1R(1)", "—/3R(4)", etc.

Experience using the Stockholm classification has shown that there is still a problem with the frequency of attacks because a minority of patients may influence the history through faulty recall or by use of protective procedures, including avoidance of cold exposure. Being history-based, the severity may be over-emphasized when compensation is being claimed. The sophisticated vascular tests (see Chapter 5) are now able to stage severity with greater accuracy, so more reliance is now being placed on them than the subjects history for staging. A scale proposed by Rigby and Cornish,[11] and developed by Griffin,[12] based on scores for the blanching of different phalanges (Figure 3-1) is available. This system has not been widely adopted, however, because only the sum score of the two hands is taken into account, and the method does not differentiate between the thumb and the other digits despite the fact that only in a small minority of cases is the thumb involved in the attacks of blanching. Furthermore it was found that the staging according to digit scores did not discriminate between stages 2 and 3 of the Taylor-Pelmear classification.[13]

Because of sluggish peripheral blood flow, some subjects demonstrate cyanosis on exposure to cold rather than frank blanching, and many subjects with cold hands have blotchy discoloration (pink, blue, and white) of the digits and palms of the hands. Intermittent or permanent cyanosis, rather than blanching attacks, follows

TABLE 3-3   The Stockholm Workshop Scale for the Classification of Sensorineural Affects of the Hand-Arm Vibration Syndrome.

Stage[a]	Symptoms
0SN	Exposed to vibration but no symptoms.
1SN	Intermittent numbness, with or without tingling.
2SN	Intermittent or persistent numbness, reduced sensory perception.
3SN	Intermittent or persistent numbness, reduced tactile discrimination and/or manipulative dexterity.

[a]The sensorineural stage is to be established for each hand.

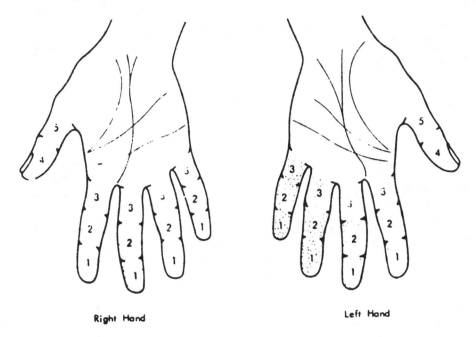

Right Hand   Left Hand

FIGURE 3-1.   Schemes for numerical scoring of digit blanching.

long-term HAV exposure when the blood supply to the tissue becomes severely depleted.

The skin of the hand is usually soft and smooth, but if there has been manual activity without gloves being worn, the skin will have callosities and fissures over the pressure points. Such skin changes may significantly impair the results of threshold measurements in sensory tests.

A small number of advanced cases (estimated at less than 1 percent) with continued HAV exposure develop peripheral trophic skin changes (fingertip ulceration). Such lesions are more common if there is an associated scleroderma.

Many subjects following initial exposure to HAV develop an edematous reaction, which is thought to be due to extrusion of fluid through the blood vessel wall because of peripheral dilatation in the early stages. Such edema causes a rise in pressure within the carpal tunnel resulting in compression on the median nerve. With prolonged exposure, secondary carpal tunnel syndrome (CTS) is not uncommon. Episodic vibratory angiodema with erythema and pruritis has also been reported.[14]

Blanching of toes from local vibration exposure may occur,[15] and recent studies have identified a higher prevalence of Raynaud's phenomenon in both fingers and toes in subjects exposed to hand or whole body vibration.[16-18] Studies indicate that the actual operation of a hand-held vibratory tool causes a reduction of skin blood flow in both the fingers and feet. The reduction in the fingers is mainly because of the combined effects of weight holding and vibration exposure, while the reduction of blood flow in the feet is mainly because of the effect of vibration exposure through the sympathetic vasoconstrictor reflex.[19-27] Studies have also shown that vibration exposure of the hand triggers sympathetic activity in the tibial nerve innervating the foot, and causes vasoconstriction of the toe and perspiration on the sole of the foot.[22]

In subjects under 45, with vascular severity no greater than stage 2, it is likely that about 30 percent will recover to stage 1 or 0 if further vibration exposure is avoided. Older subjects and those with severity stage 3, on discontinuing vibration exposure, tend to remain stationary, although some, because of atherosclerosis, continue to deteriorate. Appropriate therapy (see Chapter 6) may improve the outcome.

Neurological

Paresthesia directly after the use of a vibration tool and at night is common. It has to be distinguished from the sleep-disturbing paresthesia commonly found in CTS.[23]

Numbness, which occurs with blanching of the fingers, may persist with decreased tactile and temperature sensitivity to a lesser or greater degree between attacks in subjects more severely affected with the neurological rather than the vascular component. Impairment of skin sensory sensitivity and increased vibration perception thresholds may reflect the functional disturbance of the peripheral nerve trunks, and/or the sensory nerve endings. In some subjects the neurological symptoms predominate. They may be the presenting symptoms and result in loss of finger coordination and loss of manipulative dexterity.[24]

To stage the sensorineural effects, the Stockholm classification (Table 3-3) is now being used by most researchers and clinicians. Stage 2, which is defined as intermittent or persistent numbness, and reduced sensory perception needs to be confirmed by subjective tests for tactile, esthesiometric, and vibrotactile perception. Stage 3, intermittent or persistent numbness, reduced tactile discrimination, and/or manipulative dexterity requires additional tests and nerve-conduction evaluation (see Chapter 5).

The classification, which is applicable to individual hands, includes only those symptoms believed to be dominated by cutaneous afferent involvement.

In addition to tactile, vibrotactile, and thermal threshold impairment, a reduction in sweating of the palms may also be complained of by some subjects.

Bone, Joints and Muscles

There are many reports of *cyst formation* in the carpal bones of vibration-exposed workers.[25-29] This is a common finding in manual workers. Any increase in bone cyst formation has not yet been shown to be directly due to vibration. Bone cysts occur because of synovial fluid extrusion from joints and not from reduced blood flow. While some researchers have reported statistical differences between the vibration-exposed and controls, the statistical difference is not apparent when the controls are carefully selected as manual workers.[30-32] Gemne and Saraste[33] conducted a literature evaluation of the radiological documentation of bone and joint pathology in the hands and arms of workers using vibratory tools. They concluded that the contention that HAV causes an excess prevalence of bone cysts, vacuoles, Kienbock's disease pseudoarthrosis of the scaphoid had not been validated. They also concluded that the observed large variation in the prevalence of skeletal disorders may be explained by biodynamic and ergonomic differences between various occupations.

Osteoarthritis of the metacarpo-trapezoid joint of the thumb is sometimes noted in HAV-exposed workers, but is usually associated with tool use transmitting impact vibration to the thumb.

Kienbock's disease, because it is a sequel to disruption of the blood supply, is of particular interest. The lunate appears to be at risk due to either a limited intraosseous blood supply or a deficiency in the dorsal vessels. Vascular studies[34] have supported the cause as being due to repeated trauma with compression fractures and segmental interruption of the intraosseous blood supply. Stahl[35] reported that only 2 percent of horizontal lunate fractures developed Kienbock's disease, while Bekenbaugh et al.[36] reported that 72 percent of patients had evidence of fracture or fragmentation. Ribbans[37] reports the condition in an elderly woman with scleroderma and Raynaud's disease. He suggests that the vasculitis associated with her connective tissue disease and the increased use of her right hand was the cause. The low incidence of Kienbock's disease in HAV-exposed workers may therefore be directly due to trauma or secondary to vasospasm, but it is not yet proven.

In 67 vibration-exposed foundry workers, Bovenzi et al.[38] found that musculoskeletal symptoms, such as arthralgias of the wrist and elbow joints, muscle pain, and decreased muscular strength were found to be significantly increased in the chipping and grinding workers compared with the referents. The prevalence of cysts in the metacarpal and carpal bones was the same in the two groups, whereas radiological signs of osteoarthritis in the wrist joint were more frequent among the vibration-exposed workers. The results of this study indicate that foundry workers who used vibrating tools were affected with both bone and joint disorders in the elbow and to a lesser extent in the wrist, and these lesions occurred more frequently than was observed in unexposed referents who performed solely manual activity.

However, Malchaire et al.,[39] in a study of 82 workers using tools to quarry and slit granite blocks in stone pits, found that the prevalence of radiological changes increased markedly after the age of 45 years but was similar in the two groups, workers and controls, except for semilunar lesions, which were significantly more frequent among the exposed workers. Arthrosis in the distal radial-ulnar joint has been reported in forestry workers,[40] while in pneumatic tool users, miners, and forestry workers changes in the carpus and carpal joints—especially in the scaphoid and lunate bones—have been reported.[41] In spite of the published data there is still difficulty in attributing any bone changes to the vibratory stimulus. The interpretation of bone lesions from radiographs by different readers introduces a confounding variable.

Impairment of *grip strength* is a very common complaint in subjects who have had prolonged HAV-exposure over many years. The sensorineural staging does not include this function so it has to be evaluated separately,[42-46] and the impairment does not diminish when vibration exposure is reduced[47] or avoided. The impairment in grip strength is due to a neuromuscular fault causing incomplete muscle contraction, since muscle volume remains normal. With respect to manipulative dexterity impairment it seems that the muscular weakness may be partly due to a disturbance of the fine control of the hand muscles.[48]

High levels of *urinary hydroxyproline* excretion occur in various pathological conditions, particularly connective tissue disorders, and can be used as an index of the daily turnover of collagen in the human organism because hydroxyproline is found almost exclusively in collagen. Urinary hydroxyproline excretion is also associated with musculoskeletal system damage from the prolonged use of vibrating tools, particularly in those operators with pains in the hands and reduced grip strength.[49] In such subjects the levels are increased. That local vibration affects muscle function has also been confirmed by an increase in plasma creatinine phosphokinase (CPK) activity in rats exposed to low-frequency vibration from 30 to 480 Hz. From an analysis of the CPK isoenzymes, the increase in plasma CPK activity was shown to be due to the CPK-MM fraction originating in the skeletal muscle. The effusion of CPK from the sarcoplasm into the plasma is presumed to be due to muscular tissue destruction and a rise in permeability of the muscle cell membrane due to local vibration.[50]

Other Effects
Hearing Loss

Recent studies indicate that the hearing of subjects with HAVS may be more vulnerable to noise.[51-56] The *hearing loss* is significantly greater in subjects with HAVS who have less than 11 years vibration exposure.[57] Analysis of risk factors for the development of sensorineural hearing loss in HAV-exposed workers indicates that aging is the major risk factor, followed by exposure to occupational noise and the presence of HAVS.[58, 59] Reflex sympathetic vasoconstriction of the cochlea blood vessels is believed to cause the additional auditory vulnerability.[60] It has been noted that simultaneous exposure to HAV and *impulse* noise does not increase the risk of sensorineural hearing loss.[61]

Abdominal Injury

Leaning on vibratory tools, such as jackhammers or handles of buffing machines, while working permits low-frequency vibration to be transmitted at critical resonant frequencies (4 to 8 Hz). *Abdominal injuries* may result, including rupture of the sigmoid colon and torsion of the omentum.[62-64]

Systemic Disease

An association with scleroderma has been reported.[65] It has been suggested that exposure to HAV, in addition to the peripheral effects, may induce "Systemic disease" by causing permanent damage to the autonomic centers of the brain or causing these centers to mediate vibration stress to end organs. The symptoms could include persistent fatigue, frequent headaches, sleep disturbances, increased irritability, forgetfulness, and impotence. There is inconclusive data to confirm this hypothesis of endocrine and cardiac disfunction[66-68] other than that induced by increased sympathetic activity.[69, 70]

REPETITIVE STRAIN INJURIES

The cause and prevention of repetitive strain injuries is discussed in Chapter 8, so it will suffice to review here only the etiology and clinical picture of the more common clinical conditions.

Carpal Tunnel Syndrome (CTS)

This is the commonest entrapment neuropathy affecting the median nerve as it lies between the carpal bones, the flexor tendons, and the unyielding transverse carpal ligament (in Figure 3-2). It affects women more often than men (2 to 10 times), is most common between 30 and 50 years of age, and is bilateral in 33 percent of patients.[71]

The characteristic symptoms are nocturnal tingling and pain in the thumb, index, and middle fingers, with hypoesthesia and numbness. The paresthesia may spread to the hand and the forearm. Often the symptoms are precipitated by unaccustomed use of the hands, from exposure to HAV, or a combination of both.[72, 73] In 10 to 53 percent of patients it is secondary to other conditions including pregnancy, the premenstrual syndrome, and when the tunnel is narrowed by thickening of the synovium and flexor tendon sheaths, by tumors and deposits, or by disruption of the bony architecture. Thenar wasting is present in only 33 percent of patients.[74]

Diagnosis of CTS rests on the clinical history and use of the Tinel and Phalen provocation tests, threshold measurements of digit vibration and current perception and nerve conduction velocity. These tests are reviewed in Chapter 5.

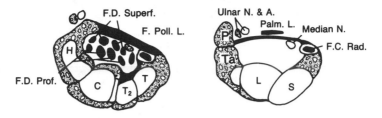

Key:

H	= Hamate	S	= Scaphoid	N = Nerve	A = Artery
C	= Capitate	L	= Lunate	F.D. Prof.	= Flexor Digitorum Profundus
T₂	= Trapezoid	Ta	= Triquetrum	F.D. Superf.	= Flexor Digitorum Sublimus
T	= Trapezium	P	= Pisiform	F. Poll. L.	= Flexor Pollicus Longus
				F.C. Rad	= Flexor Carpi Radialis
				Palm. L.	= Palmaris Longus

FIGURE 3-2.   Cross-section of wrist illustrating the relationship of the carpal bones with the nerves, arteries and tendons. The proximal part of the reinaculum is shown stretching between the scaphoid and pisiform bones, and the distal part between the trapezium and the hook of the hamate.

Dupuytren's Disease

Dupuytren's disease, a contracture of the fascial components of the lateral aspect of the palm of the hand normally affects white males over 45 years, and is usually bilateral being more advanced on one side. There is an increased incidence in association with diabetes, alcoholism, epilepsy, and it is well known to follow a single injury of the palm.[75] The association with HAV-exposure is not conclusive[76] but cases are being reported.[77]

Tenosynovitis

This inflammatory disorder of the tendon and/or sheaths may commonly follow overusage or direct trauma. It is diagnosed by swelling, tenderness, and crepitation along the affected tendon. It commonly affects the abductor pollicis longus and extensor pollicis brevis tendons of the thumb when it is known as *De Quervain's disease*. A stenosing tenosynovitis may affect any of the flexor tendons and give rise to a *trigger finger*.

SUMMARY

Hand-arm vibration syndrome has three components: vascular (circulatory), neurological (sensory and motor), and musculoskeletal disturbances (muscle weakness). The vascular effects are the most common, and the resulting blanching of the fingers is usually precipitated by cold exposure. Depending on the severity, it is graded by stage from 0 to 4. The neurological effects can develop independently and are graded stage 0 to 3. Loss of muscle power after prolonged vibration exposure is a common finding. Bone cysts are commonly reported but are not vibration induced. Other associated conditions include osteoarthritis, Keinboch's disease, CTS, Dupuytren's disease, and diffuse connective tissue disease, particularly scleroderma. Noise-induced hearing loss is reported to be significantly greater in those subjects with HAVS. Further studies are required to substantiate the synergism.

Notes

1. Gemme, G., and Taylor, W., eds. foreword. "Hand-Arm Vibration and the Central Autonomic Nervous System." In: Gemme, G., Taylor, W. eds. Special Volume. *J. Low Freq. Noise Vib.* 1983; XI.
2. Loriga, G. Pneumatic Tools. Quoted by Teleky, L. *Occup. Health Sup. ILO* 1938: 1–12.
3. Hamilton, A. "A study of Spastic Anemia in the Hands of Stonecutters. Effect of the Air Hammer on the Hands of Stonecutters." U.S. Bureau Labor Stat. 1918; 19: Bulletin 236:53–66.
4. Taylor, W., and Pelmear, P. L., eds. *Vibration White Finger in Industry*. London Academic Press, 1975: XVII–XXII.
5. Brammer, A. J.; Piercy, J. E.; Auger, P. L. "Assessment of Impaired Tactile Sensation: A Pilot Study." *Scand. J. Work. Environ. Health* 1987; 13:380–384.
6. Harada, N., and Matsumato, T. "Various Function Tests on the Upper Extremities and the Vibration Syndrome." In: Brammer, A. J., and Taylor, W., eds. *Vibration Effects on the Hand and Arm in Industry*. New York: John Wiley & Sons, 1982: 71–76.
7. Pyykkö, I.; Korhonen, O. S.; Färkkilä, M. A.; Starck, J. P.; Aatola, S. A. "A Longitudinal Study of the Vibration Syndrome in Finnish Forestry Workers." In: Brammer, A. J., and Taylor, W., eds. *Vibration Effects on the Hand and Arm in Industry*. New York: John Wiley & Sons, 1982: 157–167
8. Pyykkö, I. "Clinical Aspects of the Hand-Arm Vibration Syndrome. A Review." *Scand. J. Work. Environ. Health* 1986; 12:439–447.
9. Gemme, G.; Pyykkö, I.; Taylor, W.; Pelmear, P. L. "The Stockholm Workshop Scale for the Classification of Cold-Induced Raynaud's Phenomenon in the Hand-Arm Vibration Syndrome (Revision of the Taylor-Pelmear scale)." *Scand. J. Work. Environ. Health* 1987; 13:275–278.
10. Brammer, A. J.; Taylor, W.; Lundborg, G. "Sensorineural Stages of the Hand-Arm Vibration Syndrome." *Scand. J. Work. Environ. Health* 1987; 13:279–283.
11. Rigby, T. A., and Cornish, D. "Vibration Syndrome Research Panel." Guest Keen, and Nettlefolds (GKN Forgings Ltd.) and Rolls-Royce, Derby (England) 1984.
12. Griffin, M. J., ed. *Handbook of Human Vibration* London: Academic Press, 1990:571–575.
13. Pelmear, P. L.; Roos, J.; Leong, D.; Wong, L. "Cold Provocation Test Results From a 1985 Survey of Hard-Rock Miners in Ontario." *Scand. J. Work. Environ. Health* 1987; 13:343–347.
14. Wener, M. H.; Metzger, W. J.; Simon, R. A. "Occupationally Acquired Vibratory Angioedema With Secondary Carpal Tunnel Syndrome." *Annals Int. Med.* 1983; 98:44–46.

15. Mills, J. H. "Pneumatic Hammer Disease in Unusual Location." *Northwest Medicine* 1942; 41:282.
16. Hedlund, U. "Raynaud's Phenomenon of Fingers and Toes of Miners Exposed to Local and Whole-Body Vibration and Cold." *Int. Arch. Occup. Environ. Health* 1989; 61:457–461.
17. Sakakibara, H.; Akamatsu, Y.; Miyao, M.; Kondo, T.; Furuta, M.; Yamada, S.; Harada, N.; Miyake, S. M.; Hosokawa, M. "Correlation Between Vibration Induced White Finger and Symptoms of Upper and Lower Extremities in Vibration Syndrome." *Int. Arch. Occup. Environ Health* 1988; 60:285–289.
18. Sakakibara, H.; Hashiguchi, T.; Furuta, M.; Kondo, T.; Miyao, M.; Yamada, S. "Circulatory Disturbances of the Foot in Vibration Syndrome." *Int. Arch. Occup. Environ. Health* 1991; 63:145–148.
19. Hashiguchi, T.; Sakakibara, H.; Yamada, S. "Changes of Skin Blood Flow in the Finger and Dorsum of the Foot During Chain Saw Operation." In: Okada, A.; Taylor, W.; Dupuis, H., eds. *Hand-Arm Vibration.* Kanazawa, Japan: Kyoei Press, 1990:133–135.
20. Toibana, N. and Ishikawa, N. "Ten Patients With Raynaud's Phenomenon in Fingers and Toes Caused by Vibration." In: Okada, A., Taylor, W., Dupuis, H., eds. *Hand-Arm Vibration.* Kanazewa, Japan: Kyoei Press. 1990:245–248.
21. Sakakibara, H.; Hashiguchi, T.; Furuta, M.; Kondo, T.; Miyao, M.; Yamada, S. "Skin Temperature of the Limbs in Patients With Vibration Syndrome." In: Okada, A.; Taylor, W.; Dupuis, H., eds. *Hand-Arm Vibration.* Kanazawa, Japan: Kyoei Press, 1990:249–251.
22. Sakakibara, H.; Iwase, S.; Mano, T.; Watanabe, T.; Kobayashi, F.; Furuta, M.; Kondo, T.; Miyao, M.; Yamada, S. "Skin Sympathetic Activity in the Tibial Nerve Triggered by Vibration Applied to the Hand." *Int. Arch. Occup. Environ. Health* 1990; 62:455–458.
23. Färkkilä, M.; Koskimies, K.; Pyykkö, I.; Jäntti, V.; Starck, J.; Aatola, S.; Korhonen, O. "Carpal Tunnel Syndrome Among Forest Workers." In: Okada, A.; Taylor, W.; Dupuis, H., eds. *Hand-Arm Vibration.* Kanazawa, Japan: Kyoei Press, 1990:263–265.
24. Banister, P. A. and Smith, F. V. "Vibration-Induced White Finger and Manipulated Dexterity." *Brit. J. Ind. Med.* 1972; 29:264–267.
25. Hellstrom, B. and Andersen, K. L. "Vibration Injuries in Norwegian Forest Workers." *Brit. J. Ind. Med.* 1972; 29:255–263.
26. Kumlin, T.; Wiikeri, M.; Sumari, P. "Radiological Changes in Carpal and Metacarpal Bones and Phalanges Caused by Chain Saw Vibration." *Brit. J. Ind. Med.* 1973; 30:71–73.
27. Van den Bossche, J., and Lahaye, D. "Xray Anomalies Occurring in Workers Exposed to Vibration Caused by Eight Tools." *Brit. J. Ind. Med.* 1984; 41:137–141.
28. Laitinen, J.; Puranen, J.; Vuorinen, P. "Vibration Syndrome in Lumbermen." *J. Occup. Med.* 1974; 16:552–556.
29. Engstrom, K.; Dandanell, R.; Hammerby, S.; Lindberg, J. "Bone Changes of the Hands and Exposure Conditions Among Riveters in the Aircraft Industry." In: Okada, A.; Taylor, W.; Dupuis, H., eds. *Hand-Arm Vibration.* Kanazawa, Japan: Kyoei Press 1990:31–33.
30. James, P. B.; Yates, J. R.; Pearson, J. C. G. "An Investigation of the Prevalence of Bone Cysts in Hands Exposed to Vibration." In: Taylor, W., and Pelmear, P. L., eds. *Vibration White Finger in Industry.* New York: Academic Press, 1975:43–51.

31. Suzuki, K.; Takahashi, S.; Nakagawa, T. "Radiological Studies of the Wrist Joint Among Chain Saw Operating Lumberjacks in Japan." *Acta. Orthop. Scand.* 1978; 49:464–468.
32. Härkönen, H.; Riihimaki, H.; Tola, S.; Mattsson, T.; Pekkarinen, M.; Zitting, A.; Husman, K. "Symptoms of Vibration Syndrome and Radiographic Findings in the Wrists of Lumberjacks." *Brit. J. Ind. Med.* 1984; 41:133–136.
33. Gemme, G., and Saraste, H. "Bone and Joint Pathology in Workers Using Hand-Held Vibratory Tools—an Overview." *Scand. J. Work. Environ. Health* 1987; 13:290–300.
34. Gelberman, R. H.; Bouman, T. D.; Menon, J.; Akeson, W. H. "The Vascularity of the Lunate Bone and Kienboch's disease." *J. Hand Surg.* 1990; 5(3):272–278.
35. Strahl, F. "On Lunatomalacia (Kienbock's Disease), a Clinical and Roentgenologic Study, Especially on its Pathogenesis and the Late Results of Immobilisation Treatment." *Acta. Chirurgica Scand. Supplementum* 1947; 126:1–133.
36. Beckenbaugh, R. D.; Shives, T. C.; Dobyns, J. H.; Linscheid, R. L. "Keinbock's Disease: The Natural History of Keinbock's Disease and Consideration of Lunate Fractures." *Clinical Orthopaedics and Related Research* 1980; 149:98–106.
37. Ribbans, W. J. "Kienbock's Disease: Two Unusual Cases." *J. Hand Surg.* 1988; 13B(4):463–465.
38. Bovenzi, M.; Fiorito, A.; Volpe, C. "Bone and Joint Disorders in the Upper Extremities of Chipping and Grinding Operators." *Int. Arch. Occup. Environ.* 1987; 59:189–198.
39. Malchaire, J.; Maldague, B.; Huberlant, J. M.; Croquet, F. "Bone and Joint Changes in the Wrists and Elbows and Their Association With Hand and Arm Vibration." *Ann. Occup. Hyg.* 1986; 30(4):461–468.
40. Suzuki, K.; Takahashi, S.; Nakagawa, T. "Radiological Studies of the Wrist Joint Among Chain Saw Operating Lumberjacks in Japan." *Acta. Orthop. Scand.* 1978; 49:464–468.
41. Carlsoo, S. "The Effect of Vibration on the Skeleton, Joints and Muscles: A Review of the Literature." *Applied Ergonomics* 1982; 13(4):251–258.
42. Färkkilä, M. "Grip Force in Vibration Disease." *Scand. J. Work. Environ. Health* 1978; 4:159–166.
43. Färkkilä, M.; Pyykkö, I.; Korhonen, O.; Starck, J. "Vibration Induced Disease in the Muscle Force in Lumberjacks." *Env. J. Appl. Physiol.* 1980; 43:1–9.
44. Färkkilä, M.; Pyykkö, I.; Korhonen, O.; Stark, J. "Hand Grip Forces During Chain Saw Operation and Vibration Induced Finger in Lumberjacks." *Brit. J. Ind. Med.* 1979; 36:336–341.
45. Färkkilä, M.; Pyykkö, I.; Starck, J.; Korhonen, O. "Hand Grip Force and Muscle Fatigue in the Etiology of the Vibration Syndrome." In: Brammer, A. J., and Taylor, W., eds. *Vibration Effects of the Hand Arm in Industry.* London: John Wiley and Sons, 1983:45–50.
46. Pyykkö, I.; Korhonen, O.; Färkkilä, M.; Starck, J.; Aatola, S.; Jäntti, V. "Vibration Syndrome Among Finnish Forest Workers, a Follow-up From 1972 to 1983." *Scand. J. Work. Environ. Health* 1986; 12:307–312.
47. Färkkilä, M.; Aatola, S.; Stark, J.; Korhonen, O.; Pyykkö, I. "Hand-Grip Force in Lumberjacks: Two-Year Follow-up." *Int. Arch. Occup. Environ. Health* 1986; 58:203–208.

48. Ibid.
49. Kasamatsu, T.; Miyashita, K.; Shiomi, S.; Iwata, H. "Urinary Excretion of Hydroxyproline in Workers Occupationally Exposed to Vibration." *Brit. J. Ind. Med.* 1982; 39:173-178.
50. Okada, A.; Okuda, H.; Inaba, R.; Arhzumi, M. "Influence of Local Vibration on Plasma Creatine Phosphokinase (CPK) Activity." *Brit. J. Ind. Med.* 1985; 42:678-681.
51. Pyykkö, I.; Starck, J.; Färkkilä, M.; Hoikkala, M.; Korhonen, O.; Nurminen, M. "Hand-Arm Vibration in the Aetiology of Hearing Loss in Lumberjacks." *Brit. J. Ind. Med.* 1981; 38:281-289.
52. Iki, M.; Kurumatani, N.; Moriyama, T. "Vibration-Induced White Fingers and Hearing Loss." *Lancet* 1983:282-283.
53. Iki, M.; Kurumatani, N.; Hirata, K.; Moriyama, T. "An Association Between Raynaud's Phenomenon and Hearing Loss in Forestry Workers." *Am. Ind. Hyg. Assoc. J.* 1985; 46(9):509-513.
54. Iki, M.; Kurumatani, N.; Hirata, K.; Moriyama, T.; Satoh, M.; Arai, T. "Association Between Vibration-Induced White Finger and Hearing Loss in Forestry Workers." *Scand. J. Work. Environ. Health* 1986; 12:365-370.
55. Miyakita, T.; Miura, H.; Futatsuka, M. "Noise-Induced Hearing Loss in Relation to Vibration-Induced White Finger in Chain Saw Workers." *Scand. J. Work. Environ. Health* 1987; 13:32-36.
56. Iki, M.; Kurumatani, N.; Satoh, M.; Matsuura, F.; Arai, T.; Ogata, A.; Moriyama, T.; "Hearing of Forest Workers With Vibration Induced White Finger: A Five Year Follow Up. *Int. Arch. Occup. Environ. Health* 1989; 61:437-442.
57. Pelmear, P. L.; Leong, D.; Wong, L.; Roos, J.; Pike, M. "Hand-Arm Vibration Syndrome and Hearing Loss in Hard Rock Miners." *J. Low Freq. Noise Vib.* 1987; 6(2):49-66.
58. Pyykkö, I.; Pekkarinen, J.; Starck, J. "Sensory-Neural Hearing Loss During Combined Noise and Vibration Exposure." *Int. Arch. Occup. Environ. Health* 1987; 59:439-454.
59. Pyykkö, I.; Koskimies, K.; Starck, J.; Pekkarinen, J.; Färkkilä, M.; Inaba, R. "Risk Factors in the Genesis of Sensorineural Hearing Loss in Finnish Forestry Workers." *Brit. J. Ind. Med.* 1989; 46:439-446.
60. Iki, M.; Kurumatani, N.; Moriyama, T.; Ogata, A. "Vibration-Induced White Finger and Auditory Susceptibility to Noise Exposure." *Kurume Med. J.* 1990; 37:33-34.
61. Starck, J.; Pekkarinen, J.; Pyykkö, I. "Impulse Noise and Hand Arm Vibration in Relation to Sensory Neural Hearing Loss." *Scand. J. Work. Environ. Health* 1988; 14:265-271.
62. Kron, M. A. and Ellner, J. J. "Buffer's Belly." *N. Eng. J. Med.* 1988; 318 (9):584.
63. Shields, P. G. and Chase, K. H. "Primary Torsion of the Omentum in a Jackhammer Operator: Another Vibration Related Injury." *J. Occup. Med.* 1988; 30 (II):892-894.
64. Wasserman, D. "Jackhammer Usage and the Omentum." *J. Occup. Med.* 1989; 31 (6):563.
65. Pelmear, P. L.; Roos, J. D.; Maehle, W. M. "Occupationally induced Scleroderma." *JOM* 1992; 34 (1):21-25.
66. Gemne, Taylor eds., "Hand-Arm Vibration."
67. Färkkilä, M.; Pyykkö, I.; Heinonen, E. "Vibration Stress and the Autonomic Nervous System. *Kurume Med. J.* 1990; 37:53-60.

68. Virokannas, H. "Cardiovascular Reflexes in Workers Exposed to Hand-Arm Vibration." *Kurume Med. J.* 1990; 37:101–107.
69. Bovenzi, M. "Autonomic Stimulation and Cardiovascular Reflex Activity in the Hand-Arm Vibration Syndrome." *Kurume Med. J.* 1990; 37:85–94.
70. Olsen, N. "Hyperreactivity of the Central Sympathetic Nervous System in Vibration-Induced White Finger." *Kurume Med. J.* 1990; 37:109–116.
71. Hodgkin, K. *Towards Earlier Diagnosis.* London: Churchill Livingstone, 1973:246.
72. Wieslander, G.; Norback, D.; Gothe, C. J.; Juhlin, L. "Carpal Tunnel Syndrome (CTS) and Exposure to Vibration, Repetitive Wrist Movements, and Heavy Manual Work: A Case-Referent Study." *Brit. J. Ind. Med.* 1989; 46:43–47.
73. Koskimies, K.; Färkkilä, M.; Pyykkö, I., et al. "Carpal Tunnel Syndrome in Vibration Disease." *Brit. J. Ind. Med.* 1990; 47:411–416.
74. Heywood, P. L. "Through the Carpal Tunnel" (Editorial). *Brit. Med. J.* 1987; 294:660–661.
75. McFarlane, R. M. "Dupuytren's Contracture." In: Green, D., ed. *Operative Hand Surgery.* New York: Churchill Livingston, 1988; 608–616.
76. McFarlane, R. M. "Dupuytren's Disease: Relation to Work and Injury." *J. Hand Surg.* 1991; 16A(5):775–778.
77. Roberts, F. P. "A Vibration Injury: Dupuytrens Contracture." *J. Soc. Occup. Med.* 1981; 31:148–150.

4

Pathophysiology and Pathogenesis of Disorders in Workers Using Hand-Held Vibrating Tools

G. Gemne

This chapter concentrates on those pathogenic mechanisms for which there is sufficient documentation or a possible physiological foundation. In order not to lengthen the text unduly, a critical evaluation of each of the very many reports available has not been made. For the same reason, common clinical experience, basic physiological knowledge, and elementary requirements for epidemiologic validity have not been referenced. Especially where epidemiologic evidence is lacking, a summary statement to that effect has been made without attempting to report all pertinent references.

Pathogenic mechanisms for hand-arm vibration induced disorders are target specific, that is, the vibrations must reach an organ system in an amount sufficient to cause harmful effects. What organs or organ systems may be involved in vibration damage? The properties of vibration transmission and absorption in the hand and arm are such that they may allow vibration to cause damage to the peripheral circulation, sensory nerve structures of the hand, and parts of the locomotor apparatus of the hand and arm. The current nomenclature denoting the summation of these disturbances has been designated as the hand-arm vibration syndrome. (HAVS)[1]

Very little epidemiological work identifying the pathogenic mechanisms causing the various HAVS manifestations has been done to date. Most of our data comes from cross-sectional studies, unfortunately often with subject-selection methods that introduce bias and with disregard for various confounding factors or effect modifiers. Another source of uncertainty—perhaps the most important of all—is that there is a wide variation in individual susceptibility to damage from vibration, the nature of which is unknown. Available evidence will be analyzed and discussed for each of the target systems involved.

THE PERIPHERAL CIRCULATION

Finger skin tissue is approximately two millimeters in thickness. Vibration from hand-held tools such as grinders and chain-saws, as well as a substantial part of the energy of vibration from percussive tools, is largely absorbed in the skin where it has the potential of causing mechanical damage to blood vessels and vaso-regulatory nerve structures.

Raynaud's Phenomenon—Nature of the Lesion

The only circulatory disturbance that has been seriously considered to result from HAV exposure is the syndrome termed "vibration white fingers" (VWF) or "vibration-induced Raynaud's phenomenon." In the discussion of the localization of the lesion producing this disorder, the vascular and vasomotor nerve structures in the finger skin have been implicated and the autonomic vaso-regulatory system in general, especially its sympathetic part. The input of signals from the skin of the hand arising from vibration is believed to disturb the balance between various autonomic mechanisms to produce a net increase in sympathetic signals to the vaso-regulatory effectors: the smooth muscle cells of the vessel wall.

Vibration-Induced Sympathetic Hyperactivity
An abnormal, general elevation of sympathetic activity (termed either hyperactivity, hyper-reactivity, or over-reactivity) as the major cause of Raynaud's phenomenon in vibration-exposed workers has been strongly advocated by Olsen.[2] In a recent paper, however, the same author[3] sees this as only one of several possible mechanisms leading to vibration-induced Raynaud's phenomenon.

White fingers are said to be "basically caused by a closure of all proper digital arteries" due to "a transient vasoconstriction—predominately mediated by central sympathetic reflex mechanisms." This is seen as a manifestation of "hyper-reactivity," induced by "an activation, over a long time of vibration exposure, of central sympathetic reflex mechanisms."

The "episodic arterial closure" is also said to be either "active" (mediated by "local, humoral or central sympathetic reflex mechanisms") or "passive" (thromboembolism in a vessel with damaged endothelium, or changes in the viscoelastic properties of the arterial wall and its response to cold). The active mechanism of digital artery closure mediated by central sympathetic reflexes is seen as predominant, but other active as well as passive mechanisms, such as "abnormal adrenergic receptor activity of the smooth muscle cell" or hypertrophy of vascular smooth muscle cells, are also envisaged to contribute to some extent. This picture attempts to include all plausible mechanisms, local and humoral (residing in the finger) as well as central. A quantitative evaluation of the relative roles of these possible abnormalities was considered difficult or impossible at present. Thus, the single idea of overactive sympathetic vasoconstrictor signals as being responsible for VWF seems to have been abandoned.

These opinions, quoted from Olsen, actually summarize quite well the current multifaceted view of the nature and localization of the lesion, the details of which will be discussed later.

Autonomic Dysfunction and Hemodynamic Changes Connected With Stressors

Several researchers have reported that the prevalence of signs of sympathetic hyperactivity (affecting not only the peripheral circulation in the form of white fingers but also cardiac functions) is higher in vibration-exposed subjects than in nonexposed controls. Vibration as one of many possible stressors has been postulated to cause such changes.

Thus, in a study of forestry workers with VWF, Färkkilä et al.[5] regarded the orthostatic hypotension that they observed as a sign of "autonomic failure," similar to the autonomic failure from other causes.[6] The symptoms and signs resembled those induced by mental and physical stress.[7] It was not stated whether symptoms were to be considered permanent or chronic. The lesion behind the VWF in the lumberjacks was considered to be at the afferent side of the sympathetic nervous system, because the vasoconstrictor response to stressors was found to predominate.

Bovenzi,[8] in an investigation of grinders, and Heinonen et al.[9] in a study of chain-saw workers, did not explicitly mention stressors as etiologic factors, but the effects of the vibration exposure were of the same kind as in the study by Färkkilä and collaborators previously mentioned. Bovenzi recorded blood pressure, heart rate and systolic time intervals in response to a battery of typical "stress" tests for sympathetic tone. From the results, for instance, of systolic time intervals, he concluded that excessive sympathetic reflex activity plays an important role in the pathogenesis of VWF. A vibration-induced autonomic dysfunction was also discussed in the report of Heinonen and co-workers. In their investigation, however, an enhancement of sympathetic vasomotor tone was postulated to result from a depression of parasympathetic activity. Similar interpretations were made by Harada et al.,[10] discussed in a later section.

In summary, the theory of stressor-induced sympathetic hyperfunction causing autonomic disturbances, including white fingers and psychosomatic symptoms, has the advantage of not having to reckon with damage to the central nervous system. Instead it is founded on a more simple and plausible physiological mechanism. In some individuals, the stressor effect only consists of an imbalance between different components of the autonomic cardiovascular efferent system. The degree of chronicity of these effects has not been clarified. Further research in this field should be given priority. In some particularly susceptible individuals, stress from vibration and other factors may result in psychosomatic manifestations. These seem to be very rare.

Relationship to Primary Raynaud's Phenomenon

Primary Raynaud's phenomenon (PRP, also called Raynaud's disease) is defined[11] as attacks of finger skin vasoconstriction triggered by cold or emotion in subjects without any known cause or associated pathological conditions. When there is a likely etiology, such as trauma, or the subject suffers from systemic and other disorders where Raynaud's phenomenon may occur (such as arteriosclerosis, diabetes, scleroderma, obliterating thromboangiitis, or symptoms associated with drug therapy) we speak of secondary Raynaud's phenomenon (SRP). Studies on Raynaud's phenomenon often do not make a distinction between the subjects with regard to possible underlying conditions.

Secondary Raynaud's Phenomenon, according to definition, includes VWF as a subgroup. Primary Raynaud's Phenomenon, as well as most nonvibration SRP, differs symptomatologically from VWF in that the typical appearance of PRP is considered mostly to be a bilateral, diffuse blanching of most fingers of both hands. Although this is certainly not always the case, the contrast to the more patchlike distribution of the blanching in VWF is nevertheless clear. Can something be derived from studies of PRP? Yes, possibly, but extrapolation of the findings to VWF patients cannot readily be made.

The blood pressure in individuals with PRP or SRP other than VWF may be somewhat lower than normal.[12] This would explain the increased tendency to experience attacks of white fingers, since low blood pressure facilitates arterial closure in the cold. However, no difference in blood pressure between persons with and without VWF has been demonstrated in epidemiological studies.

In patients with PRP, sympathetic hyperactivity has not been unequivocally demonstrated. Significant sympathetic contribution to PRP seems to have been logically derived from the fact that the diagnostic sensitivity of finger systolic blood pressure during local cooling can be increased by simultaneous cooling of the whole body.[13, 14] Coffman and Cohen[15] found that finger blood flow in a warm environment was lower in patients with PRP than in normal subjects, indicating a hyperactivity of sympathetic vasoconstrictor activity.

In another study on PRP subjects, however, plethysmographic recordings from the fingers of one hand failed to show any reflex sympathetic vasoconstriction in response to local cooling of the contralateral hand.[16] In microelectrode recordings from single median nerve fibers on one hand while cooling the other,[17] the cold-induced increase in nerve activity of patients with PRP did not differ from that of normal subjects. Elevated urinary or plasma catecholamine levels have not been demonstrated in subjects with PRP.[18]

Lewis[19] found support for a "local fault" (that is, a lesion in the finger skin) in PRP patients in the fact that attacks of skin blanching could be provoked by cold in single fingers with intact nerve supply as well as in sympathetically enervated fingers.

The symptoms in patients with some types of SRP (with associated pathological conditions) can be alleviated by treatment with calcium antagonists.[20, 21] This indicates the existence of a lesion in the endothelium and/or the smooth muscle cells of the vessel wall. There are no reports or reliable results of this kind in subjects with VWF. The mechanical influence from vibrations may very well have produced a specific kind of injury to the endothelium that does not involve calcium-dependent functions.

That a local factor is involved is supported by an experiment[22] where local application of rapidly decompressed nitrogen on the nailfold elicited an arrest of blood flow in 88 percent of subjects with PRP but only in 15 percent of the controls.

Cyanotic discoloration as a feature of the vasoconstrictive attack in PRP patients may signify an etiologic contribution from arteriosclerosis.[23]

Localization of the Lesion to the Finger

Strong evidence from experimental studies has accumulated for the assumption that the decisive lesion behind VWF resides in the finger skin rather than being sympathetic overactivity. The latter mechanism is, for instance, not consistent with such differentiated manifestations as vasospasm in one part, and only a general pallor of the skin or normal hue in the rest of the finger. In typical cases,[24] the distribution of finger skin blanching corresponds to the parts of the hand that have been most strongly exposed to vibration, and the blanched areas are distinctly demarcated from surrounding, normal skin. The proposition that the cold-provoked SRP in *individual* fingers is the result of vasospasm in (some, but obviously not all) digital arteries also seems to require the presence of a local disturbance.

Spasm in Digital Arteries

Experiments involving measurement of finger systolic blood pressure (FSBP, as measured with a sphygmomanometer around the finger) during local finger and general body cooling[25] have shown[26] that FSBP is very low in a large proportion of VWF patients. It was concluded on the basis of indirect evidence that the primary mechanism producing the blanching is a closure of the two digital arteries of the affected fingers.

The idea of an obligatory digital artery spasm appears to be in conflict with the fact that typical VWF as well as other SRP occur in well-demarcated patches of the finger skin, which may not always extend over the whole width of the finger. A white patch may even be localized proximal to an unaffected skin area.

The credibility of a closure of the digital arteries (Figure 4-1) as the sole mechanism behind the blanching thus seems questionable. The conclusion, instead, must be that, for the white finger patch to appear, a closure of the digital artery terminal branches and/or of the arterioles of the capillary loops is required (Figure 4-2). If the theory of digital artery spasm is not the only or major explanation for white fingers, then the FSBP recordings previously mentioned may not always tell the full story.

Endothelial Damage—Functional Adrenergic Receptor Changes

Recent extension of our knowledge of endothelial mechanisms governing peripheral circulation[27] has led to a natural focusing of interest on receptors and functions in the endothelium of the vessel wall as plausible targets for harmful effects of HAV. The endothelial vaso-regulatory mechanisms are numerous and complexly inter-related. Damage to the endothelium might result in changes in vasomotor functions that require an intact vessel wall. A defect in the release of endothelial vasodilators or a modification of their effect on smooth muscle cells might then result.

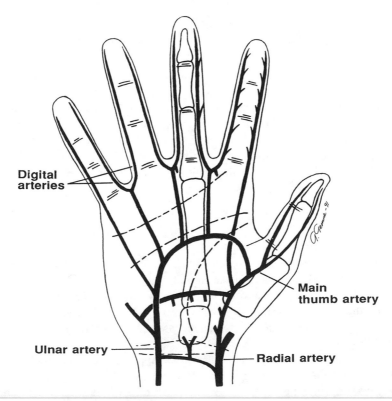

FIGURE 4-1.   The digital artery circulation.

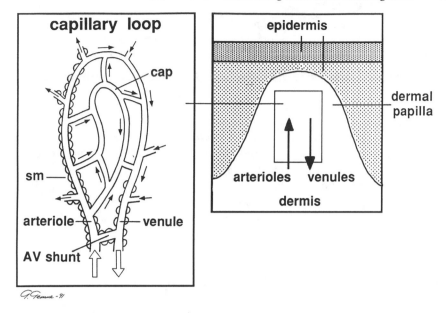

FIGURE 4-2.   Capillary loops in dermal papillae (sm = smooth muscle; cap = capillary).

The damaging mechanism may be mechanical in nature, but other factors in the working environment, such as cold, may contribute. In man, no evidence has been produced for the pathogenic importance of cold, but some indication comes from animal experimentation. Endrich[28] reported on extensive endothelial damage, as seen by electron microscopy, in capillaries and venules (but not in arterioles) of a dorsal skin fold in hamsters exposed to nonfreezing cold for five consecutive days.

Experiments by Jamieson et al.,[29] were interpreted to show that the enhanced reflex sympathetic vasoconstriction in patients with PRP or scleroderma in response to local hand cooling is mediated by cold-sensitized vasoconstrictor alpha-adrenergic receptors on smooth muscle cells.

Interesting observations on adrenergic functions in the finger skin have been made in studies where vasoactive substances were administered to the finger skin by iontophoresis:

1. In an experiment on 12 VWF patients and as many healthy controls not exposed to vibration, Ekenvall and Lindblad[30] recorded the response of finger blood flow to noradrenaline (NA, stimulating vasoconstrictor alpha-1 and alpha-2 receptors), phenylephrine (PE, alpha-1 agonist) and B-HT 933 (alpha-2 agonist). There was no group difference for NA and B-HT 933, while the reaction of the patients to PE was significantly weaker than that of the controls. The suggestion from these findings was that Raynaud's phenomenon in

persons damaged by vibration may be due to a selective damage to alpha-1 receptors, resulting in abnormally strong vasoconstrictor response to *skin cooling*. This reasoning was founded on the interpretation by Vanhoutte et al.[31] of earlier observations[32] that cooling affects alpha-2 receptors more than alpha-1 receptors to produce an increase in NA-triggered vasoconstriction.

2. A study of finger skin blood flow during local cooling was performed on ten healthy industrial workers.[33] Cold-induced vasoconstriction was abolished after iontophoretic administration of rauwolscine, an alpha-2 adrenoceptor antagonist, but not after the alpha-1 antagonist, doxazosin. In another study,[34] vasoconstriction provoked in six VWF patients by local finger skin cooling was abolished by rauwolscine. The results of these two studies were interpreted to indicate that vasoconstriction on local cooling in the human finger skin is mainly mediated by alpha-2 adrenoreceptors and that substances inhibiting them may be of therapeutic value in patients with VWF.

The alpha-2 receptor has also been implicated as the one responsible for cold-induced constriction of human *veins*.[35] The contractile response to cooling *in vitro* of cutaneous vein segments obtained from 50 patients without vascular disorders (16 of whom were men) was investigated using agonists and antagonists to specifically study the functions of alpha-1 and alpha-2 receptors respectively. A great variability between individuals was observed in the relative distribution of the two receptor types. Cooling to 25°C most often caused contraction of vessels mediated by alpha-2 receptors but relaxation of those vessels where alpha-1 receptors predominated. It was concluded that alpha-2 antagonist substances might be of therapeutic interest in order to relieve vasospasm in the hand vessels.

A few remarks are appropriate here to illuminate the complexity of adrenergic mechanisms involved in skin vasoregulation (Figure 4-3). Norepinephrine (NE) contracts smooth muscle by acting on alpha-adrenoceptors and consequent stimulation of calcium utilization (facilitation of calcium entry and of calcium release from the sarcoplasmic reticulum). However, NE has also a negative feedback on alpha-2 adrenoceptors localized on the sympathetic varicosity. Furthermore, inhibition of NE release is induced by prostaglandin, as well as through muscarinic receptors[36]. A smooth muscle relaxing effect of catecholamines is produced by epinephrine acting on beta-2 adrenoceptors: inhibition of calcium entry, stimulation of adenylate cyclase and cAMP, and decrease of calcium utilization by the smooth muscle cells.

If veins do indeed participate in the elicitation of Raynaud's phenomenon, then yet another system may be of great importance, namely the serotonergic receptor functions. In *in vitro experiments* on vein segments from the human hand,[37] ketanserin—an antagonist of 5-hydroxytryptamine (5-HT, serotonin)—diminished the cold-induced enhancement of vasoconstriction mediated by 5-HT_2 receptors.

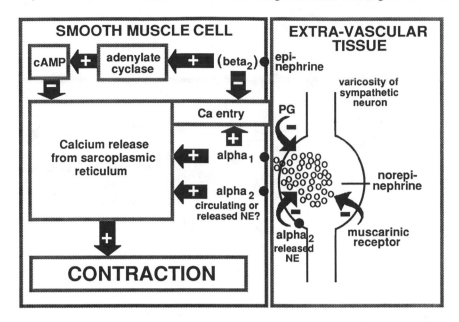

FIGURE 4-3.   Schematic representation of the adrenergic system involved in skin vasoregulation.

The intricacy of the serotonergic system and its associated mechanisms is no less considerable (Figure 4-4). Platelet aggregation leads to the release of serotonin. Besides promoting further release of 5-HT from the platelets, serotonin also induces endothelium-derived relaxing factor (EDRF) and prostacyclin release from the endothelial cells. These substances, by way of inhibiting platelet aggregation and relaxing smooth muscle, contribute to vasodilation. A delicate balance between smooth muscle contraction and relaxation is produced by these mechanisms.

The vascular response to *cold* is complex.[38] In addition to the general diversity of interacting receptor systems (adrenergic, cholinergic, and serotonergic), there are several subtypes of specific receptors.[39, 40] The differential distribution and functional significance of these various receptor types are still largely unknown. It is clear that differences in receptor population determine the effect of cooling.

The interplay between various vasoregulatory systems in response to cold is illustrated in Figure 4-5. Vasoactive mechanisms residing in the endothelium of the vessel wall play an important role in vasodilatation. Acetycholine (and its agonist, metacholine) acting through the muscarine receptors on the endothelial cell stimulates EDRF (which is probably nitric oxide) and causes smooth muscle relaxation. Nitric oxide (NO) as well as the agonists, nitroprusside and nitroglycerine, release prostacyclin (prostaglandin I_2) with the same smooth muscle effect. This process involves stimulation of adenylate and guanylate cyclases which increase the

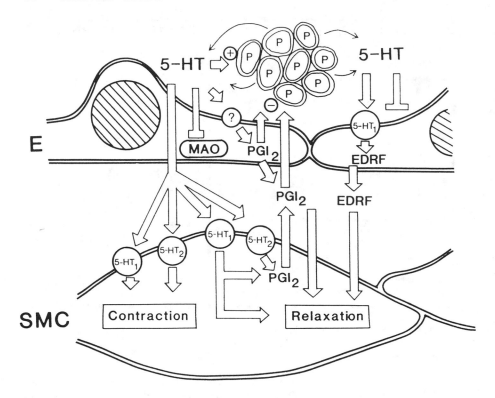

FIGURE 4-4.   Interactions between platelets (P), endothelium (E), and smooth muscle cells (SMC) involving serotonin (5-HT). EDRF = endothelium-derived relaxing factor; MAO = monoamine oxidase (metabolizing some of the serotonin). PGI_2 = prostaglandin I_2 (prostacyclin). 5-HT1 and 5-HT2 = different types of serotonin receptors. (Reproduced with permission from Bodelsson 1990[38].)

activity of cyclic GMP and AMP to inhibit calcium utilization for smooth muscle contraction. Nitric oxide also acts directly to contract smooth muscle.

The results of recent experiments[41] with iontophoresis of sodium nitroprusside and metacholine into the finger skin of chain-sawyers and laser-Doppler recording of blood flow suggests that vibration exposure may damage endothelial vasoregulatory mechanisms. A weaker vasodilatory reaction to metacholine, but not to nitroprusside, was observed in the combined group of subjects with current and past white finger than in those who had never experienced the syndrome. This agrees with the physiological premises (Figure 4-4): metacholine induces relaxation only through EDRF, while nitroprusside also has direct access to the smooth muscle. Thus, the results are consistent with endothelial damage and disturbance of the EDRF-mediated vasodilatory function.

Cold, as well as vessel-wall injury, causes platelet aggregation and skin vasoconstriction as a net effect of the liberation of various vasoactive substances.[42]

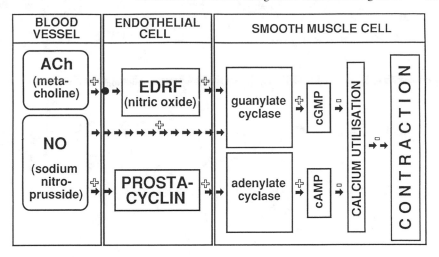

BLOOD VESSEL	ENDOTHELIAL CELL	SMOOTH MUSCLE CELL

FIGURE 4-5.   Endothelial vasoactive mechanisms.

A conclusion to be drawn from the studies presented here is that, in experimentation on humans, it is difficult to control the several mechanisms operating simultaneously in response to cold stimulation of the skin. All theories hitherto advanced concerning the pathophysiology of VWF should therefore be regarded with scepticism.

·Myogenic Versus Neurogenic Control of Blood Flow in VWF

Fluctuation in blood flow (vasomotor oscillation) is a physiologically normal feature in small arteries involved in the kinetics of capillary exchange. In laser-Doppler flux recordings from the finger skin under controlled thermal conditions,[43] such fluctuations were studied in six men with VWF and ten healthy controls. The results indicated that, whereas the myogenic component of vasomotor activity was essentially the same in both groups, the mechanism of neurogenic control of vasomotor tone was weaker in subjects with VWF. This may suggest the existence of autonomic neuropathy localized in the finger skin.

Anatomical Changes in the Skin Vessels

A patho-anatomical mechanism has been proposed that does not require sympathetic hyperactivity, namely a reduction in the bore of the skin blood vessels in VWF subjects because of either hypertrophy of the vessel wall smooth muscle layer and/or intimal thickening.[44, 45] If the smooth muscle layer of the vessel is hypertrophic (Figure 4-6), a normal contraction in response to cold may result in a lumen decrease strong enough to cause Raynaud's phenomenon.[46] This result may also ensue in vessels with a smooth muscle layer of normal thickness, provided that other pathophysiological mechanisms have caused the contraction to be abnor-

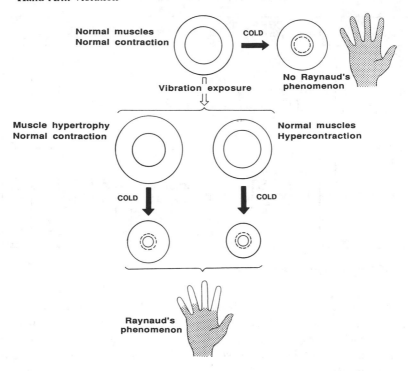

FIGURE 4-6.   Antomical and physiological mechanisms of lumen reduction. (Reproduced with permission from Gemne 1982[45].)

mally strong. In both these alternatives, a proportionately greater reduction of blood flow would be the result of normal sympathetic activity.

It is possible that repeated dilation and constriction of a skin blood vessel over a long time, caused by various stimuli present in the working environment of a person using vibrating tools, could result in smooth muscle cell hypertrophy. Walton[47] reported in a case of Raynaud's phenomenon of occupational origin that in some sections the digital arteries showed marked media hypertrophy and fibrosis, with reduction of the lumen by extensive intimal proliferation and elastosis. In biopsies from 60 fingers of VWF patients, examined with light microscopy, Takeuchi et al.[48] found that in each case there was a thickening of the muscular layers of the arteries because of hypertrophy of individual muscle cells. In addition, there was a destruction of myelin sheaths and fewer nerve fibres in 73 percent of the biopsies. Intimal thickening has been discussed as a possible sequel of vibration exposure[49, 50] according to a theory involving growth and migration of smooth muscle cells to the intima.[51]

A statistically significant elevation in whole blood viscosity (but not in plasma viscosity) has been observed in vibration-exposed subjects with VWF compared with those without.[52] The difference was independent of age and duration of vibration exposure. In rats whose hind legs had been vibration-exposed at 60 Hz and 50 m/s² 4 hours a day for 90 days,[53] whole blood viscosity was higher than in a nonexposed control group. Intimal thickening was also observed in the rats, and the viscosity increase was tentatively related to concomitant vessel-wall damage and fibrocellular thickening of the intima. Such a mechanism was also postulated to occur in persons with VWF. A reduced vessel diameter drastically increases blood viscosity but other factors related to vessel diameter and viscosity (for instance turbulence) also strongly influence blood flow.[54] It is therefore not immediately evident what physiological significance the observations of changes in viscosity might have for the vasospasm in VWF.

Lumen reduction may cause diminished capacity to dilate the vessel in warm environmental conditions. Such a deficiency would be consistent with the results obtained in finger blood flow recordings in a climate chamber.[55] In the stage of maximal vasodilation (room temperature 45°C and anaesthesia of the digital sympathetic nerves), the arterial blood inflow in the finger after arterial occlusion with a cuff was considerably lower in the VWF subjects than in persons without Raynaud's phenomenon. A relative increase in peripheral resistance in VWF subjects[56, 57] may also be related to lumen restriction of the vessels.

It has been postulated that mechanical trauma may cause circulatory disturbances. Wegelius[58] found a higher frequency of arterial obstruction (occlusion and lumen obliteration) in stonecutters than in a control group. The findings were correlated with age and chronic trauma. There was, however, no difference in the occurrence of arterial obstruction between subjects with VWF, and age-matched subjects with hard manual work without vibration exposure. That trauma to the skin by vibration can result in local organic change has also been suggested by Arneklo-Nobin,[59] who reported a slower rewarming rate in vibration-exposed persons after finger cooling even when dilatation was enforced with oral administration of alcohol. The question whether vessel lumen reduction or functional changes or both is the main factor in the causation of reduced blood flow in VWF subjects remains to be settled.

Influence of Cold on the Development of White Fingers
An obvious clue to the pathogenesis of white fingers should be looked for in the fact that Raynaud's phenomenon is typically elicited by environmental cold, especially when the whole body is cooled. This, of course, does not necessarily make cold pathogenic, but it is at least highly possible that cold exposure contributes to the development of VWF. The characteristic reaction pattern of a VWF subject is sometimes called "cold hypersensitivity." The meaning of this term is not clear. It may be used only to indicate that cold triggers blanching attacks or it may refer to a pathophysiological mechanism operating in the finger vasculature, either as a manifestation of sympathetic hyperactivity or an enhanced response of the vasomotor

receptors (or effectors) to a cold stimulus. Individuals with a constitutional tendency to a high level of sympathetic activity can more easily than others pass the threshold where blood flow is so severely reduced that finger pallor ensues. Prolonged influence of various vasoconstrictive factors, such as vibration and cold, may also raise the level of sympathetic activity enough to cause attacks of VWF (Figure 4-7).[60]

Many persons habitually experience cold and a consequent diffuse pallor in their fingers and toes. The role of such a constitutional disposition has not been epidemiologically clarified, but it is physiologically reasonable that persons with this trait (indicating a high sympathetic activity) are more susceptible to harmful influence from various vasoconstrictor stimuli. Since the exposure to different vasoconstrictors varies widely, this explanation would also account for the great variation always observed in the prevalence of white fingers in different occupational groups.[61]

Peripheral vaso-regulation is inherently sensitive to cold. Thus, cold influences neuronal activity, receptor mechanisms, smooth muscle contractile elements, platelets, endothelial mechanisms, and rheological factors.[62] Cold triggers a whole series of events that influence the net reactivity of the system. In the absence of epidemiologic studies with successful control of these events, the question of cold as a pathogenic factor cannot be answered. It is of course suggestive that white fingers are not reported from countries with a warm climate, but this may simply be explained by the absence of symptom-triggering cold stimuli.

Relationship of Vascular to Neurological Disturbances

An interesting question is whether the diffuse neuropathy in the hand observed in many vibration-exposed persons is causally connected with Raynaud's phenome-

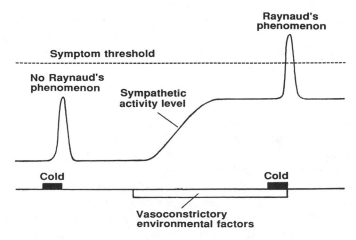

FIGURE 4-7. Influence on the level of sympathetic activity of repeated and prolonged vasoconstrictory stimulation. (Reproduced with permission from Gemme 1982[45].)

non. It is possible that sensory disturbances arise because of repeated, prolonged ischemia in the nerve structures caused by vasospastic attacks. This idea would appear to be supported by the results of Lundborg et al.,[63] who found that abnormalities in vibration perception threshold in vibration-exposed workers in various occupations correlated with the occurrence of white fingers as well as numbness and pain. Other authors have reported similar results, contrary data have also been published. For the time being, this issue remains unsettled. The vascular and neurological disturbances may well be pathogenically independent despite the fact that they both occur in the same vibration-exposed individual. Such a conclusion was drawn by Hayward and Griffin[64] in a study on metal and chain saw workers, where sensory perception threshold elevation was not restricted to finger areas showing Raynaud's phenomenon.

Relationship Between Effects of Noise and Vibration
The hearing level at particularly noise-sensitive frequencies has been shown to be lower in forestry workers with white fingers than in those without[65-77]. The pathophysiology behind this observation is unclear. To judge from the results of recent transmission measurements,[78] it is unlikely that vibration from hand-held tools is transmitted to the inner ear in amounts sufficient to cause a direct mechanical effect on cochlea structures. The sensory input from the vibration-exposed hand, however, may result in an elevation, over a prolonged period, of the sympathetic activity that produces a harmful effect on the cochlea cells by a relatively stronger vasoconstriction (and consequent ischemia) than with noise alone. Further epidemiological studies are needed to clarify this question.

Electroencephalography
Some reports have been published describing changes in EEG in vibration-exposed workers. Thus, Arikawa et al.[79], in subjects with "vibration disease" of advanced stages (Soviet classification), found an abnormality in the form of a pronounced fast activity with spindles correlated with the subjects' complaints of sleep disturbances alleged to be induced by vibration exposure. It was also said that the observations might indicate "excitation and functional impairment of the diencephalon, primarily the hypothalamus" and "alterations in the function of the ascending reticular activating system." The relation of data of this kind to vibration exposure has never been confirmed.

Koishizawa et al.[80] have reported on EEG findings in two studies. One involved 312 men with vibration syndrome and controls with headache and vertigo without organic causes, the other, 96 vibration-exposed men with and without VWF (48 unexposed healthy men as controls). In study 1, the prevalence of diffuse alpha activity was higher than in the controls. In study 2, the vibration-exposed subjects had a higher prevalence of this EEG feature than the controls, regardless of VWF. The findings indicated a slight depression in brain function, which may be related to a regional decrease in brain blood flow. The possibility of cerebral arteriosclerosis as a causative factor was not excluded. A specific relationship of the findings to vibration exposure was denied.

Hormones and Other Biochemical Substances

The question of autonomic disturbance in vibration-exposed persons has also been addressed by investigating some substances that, in an oversimplified way, have been used as biochemical indicators of sympathetic and parasympathetic activity. In the papers published so far, other physiological mechanisms have not been properly controlled. The results are therefore inconclusive.

The inherent difficulties may be exemplified by the study of Harada et al.[81] investigating 41- to 69-year old vibration-exposed men with and without VWF. After correction for age, cold exposure of the whole body was found to result in a higher rise in norepinephrine and thyroid hormones (T3 and T4) than in healthy controls. There was also a relatively greater rise in cAMP and cGMP, which was interpreted to indicate that the cold-induced response of receptors on nerve endings was enhanced in subjects with vibration syndrome. In another study,[82] a smaller variation in electrocardiographic R-R intervals in vibration-exposed men (regardless of the presence of white fingers) was taken to indicate a relative reduction of basal parasympathetic activity. A relatively greater rise of cGMP in response to cold in the vibration-exposed was interpreted as a sign of hyperfunction of sympathetic alpha-2 receptors or of parasympathetic muscarinic receptors.

Interpretations of this kind may or may not be valid. However, concerning the central question whether vibration exposure is the causative factor of the pathophysiology observed, serious doubt must be raised. Environmental and psychological confounders of the stressor type or effect-modifiers related to the individual may very well have played an important role for this "autonomic unbalance." In the work of Harada and collaborators previously mentioned,[83] subjects with VWF had not only "disturbances of upper extremities" but "various generalized symptoms" reflected in a higher Cornell Medical Index (CMI) for both physical and psychological items. It was not discussed whether the observed values of certain biochemical variables in these subjects may have been related to the influence of various stressors. For example, there is the adverse psychological reaction of the subjects who considered themselves to be damaged by vibration. The criteria for selection were not described. In many cases, persons with a constitutional predisposition to stress-induced autonomic reactions in general may also respond more strongly to experimental and clinical situations.

Susceptibility

The variation in individual susceptibility to damage from vibration is large. In occupational groups where the majority of the members have carried out essentially identical work for an equal amount of time, there is variation in the latent interval due to normal interindividual differences in susceptibility related to, for instance, the habitual width of skin vessels. Awareness of the variation has to be a major consideration in prevention. It has the important physiopathological implication that vibration may sometimes be much less etiologically significant than human factors related to the individual.

Nicotine

There is a fundamental distinction between physiological and biochemical events involved in the development of a disorder (pathogenic mechanisms) and those only connected with its manifestations (symptomatologic mechanisms). The role of smoking in VWF subjects illustrates this point. Nicotine, like cold, has a constrictory effect on blood vessels, and the peripheral blood flow of heavy smokers therefore tends to be smaller than that of nonsmokers. This results in lower skin temperatures in their fingers and toes in a cold environment. Habitual use of tobacco has been demonstrated to aggravate white finger symptoms, as shown by an increased reactivity to cold,[84] and many cross-sectional studies have demonstrated a higher VWF prevalence in smokers than in nonsmokers. Others have failed to do so.

There is little sense in reviewing the great number of these investigations that consider only current smoking, since it is obvious that they cannot decide whether nicotine is also a pathogenic factor. It is not surprising that there is yet no clear epidemiologic evidence for or against this theory. Past smoking cannot be accurately quantified because of recall bias, and there is difficulty with the estimation of exposure dose, which depends greatly on differences in inhalation habits and nicotine content of the tobacco. The difficulties involved in epidemiologic research in this area are illuminated by a study of reindeer herders in Finland.[85] The risk for white fingers in these subjects, who were exposed to vibration from snowmobile handles and chain saws, was analyzed in a logistic regression model. The WF risk was found to depend more on the lifetime amount of smoking than on current smoking, with the implicit interpretation that smoking is an etiologic factor in the development of VWF. However, vascular effects of both smoking and vibration may be subject to an age-dependent modification by cold. Since exposure to this environmental factor was not taken into account, the results, unfortunately, cannot be said to clarify the pathogenic role of smoking alone.

Age

There are several studies[86-88] demonstrating a correlation between the occurrence or severity of white fingers and age. They have, however, failed to separate in a statistically unequivocal way age from vibration-exposure duration, other environmental confounders and individual effect modifiers. Longitudinal investigations of this question have not been reported.

Vibration as an Attack Trigger? Beneficial Effects
of Vibration.

Workers exposed to HAV report Raynaud's phenomenon less frequently while actually operating their tools. One possible explanation is that the vibration energy is partly transformed into heat, which dissipates through the tissues and causes a secondary effect in the form of vasodilation. Another alternative is that the manual work necessitates an increase (elicited as a autonomic reflex) in blood supply to the fingers, which warms the skin to the extent that a cold-induced attack is effectively counteracted. Observations by Färkkilä and Pyykkö[89] in a photo-plethysmographic investigation of lumberjacks seem to support the latter assumption. In 75 percent of all trials, muscle work in the form of repeatedly gripping a handle, with or without simultaneous handle vibration, resulted in vasodilation in the finger skin of the other hand.

Vibration exposure also has a beneficial effect, which may be of some significance for the question of pathophysiological mechanisms in VWF. Although large-amplitude vibration (120 to 200μm) causes vasoconstriction (as assessed by plethysmography) in the exposed finger,[90] low-amplitude vibration (5 to 20μm) in the frequency range 150 to 300 Hz increases finger skin temperature.[91, 92] In the latter studies, the vasodilation (also occurring contralaterally) was due to a reflex inhibition of vasomotor tone by vibration-induced inflow of signals from certain mechanoreceptors.

Vasodilation in response to low-amplitude vibration also seems to be in concordance with the commonly known effect that is produced by "massage rods" and other devices advertised to relax musculature and increase blood circulation. The feeling of tension in the muscles diminishes and a sense of pleasant warmth spreads over the skin. As a possible contributory effect, the vibrations and the pressure from a massage rod moved over the skin may also relieve tension by distributing excess fluid (for instance trapped in muscle compartments) more evenly over the arm and to carry it away through lymph channels.

Vibration may interact with physiological processes relating to vaso-regulation. Ljung and Sivertsson[93] observed a dilatation of the blood vessel brought about by the vibration caused by blood flow turbulence in isolated dog veins and arteries. The effect was ascribed to the effect of vibration on the actin-myosin cross links in the vessel-wall muscle cells.

SENSORY NERVE CONDITIONS

Diffuse Neuropathy

The sensory nerve supply to the hand is mediated by the median and ulnar nerves. Their receptor structures and nerve fibers reside in the skin tissues and, like the blood vessels, therefore may be targets of harmful effects from vibration. The role of the mechanoreceptors in relation to the vibration stimulus is described in Chapter 1.

Increased prevalence of neurologic symptoms in the hand, suggestive of diffuse neuropathy induced by vibration, has often been reported, but the pathogenic mechanisms need to be further clarified. Only a few studies have addressed this question. Lundborg et al.[94] exposed the hind limb of rats to vibration at 82 Hz with peak to peak amplitude of 0.21 mm for 4 hours a day for 5 days. Edema developed in the epineurium of the sciatic nerve, possibly associated with an increase in blood vessel permeability. It was suggested that such an effect of vibration might result in nerve function disturbance through interference with "nerve fiber nutrition." The justification for extrapolation of these observations to subjects with VWF (further commented on p. 60) has not been proven. A few cross-sectional studies have been published, for instance that of Takeuchi et al.[95] In biopsies of 60 fingers from 30 patients with VWF they found demyelinating neuropathy in the peripheral nerves and perineural fibrosis, which appeared to be characteristic of VWF subjects. The interpretation of these findings was that the fibrosis was due to previous edema resulting from vibration exposure. Observations of this sort have as yet to be validated epidemiologically.

Ekenvall et al.[96] investigated 37 patients with neurologic symptoms (paresthesias, numbness, pain) in the hands. The temperature receptors are supplied with thin myelinated and unmyelinated afferent nerve fibers, and the results indicate that damage to these receptors or fibers is common in the vibration syndrome. Diffuse neuropathy, however, has a multifactorial etiology. In a study of dentists[97] exposed to high-frequency vibration from their drills, Ekenvall and collaborators found that the long-term exposed (about 20 years) group had higher vibration thresholds than a group with short exposure (about 2 years). This was so in both an exposed and an unexposed finger, whereas the temperature and pain thresholds were similar. The long-term exposed group had neurological symptoms (paresthesia) in the dominant hand more often than the short-time group. Because the vibration-exposed and nonexposed fingers were similarly affected, the interpretation was made that the sensory disturbances (which resembled those described in subjects with HAV syndrome) had been caused by factors other than vibration, for instance ergonomic conditions typical for dentistry work, such as repetitive hand grips with elbow flexion, and cervical spine flexion and rotation.

Brezinova and Quinton,[98] in an examination of 20 metal workers using pneumatic equipment, found that the abnormal nerve conduction velocities observed did not correlate with the vascular disturbances, which supports the prevailing opinion that the vascular and sensorineural components of HAVS are separate entities.

Compression Syndromes

The *median nerve* passes to the hand through the carpal tunnel of the wrist (Figures 4-8 and 4-9) together with the nine finger flexor tendons. The bottom of the tunnel consists of carpal bones, and its roof of the tough and inelastic flexor retinaculum ligament. The median nerve conducts sensory information from digits one through three, and the radial part of digit four. Compression of the median nerve causes *carpal tunnel syndrome* (CTS), which typically presents as nocturnal paresthesia with numbness and, sometimes, pain.

The extensive literature dealing with the etiology of CTS can be only briefly reviewed here. The pathogenic mechanism in this disorder may be repeated mechanical insult and compression of the nerve from the flexor tendons. Compression would also build up in the diminished tunnel space caused by inflammation in the flexor tendon synovia (synovitis) resulting from excessive flexion and extension.[99, 100] Another possible mechanism is the increased intratunnel pressure resulting from certain maintained postures of the hand and wrist that diminish the width of the tunnel. It is therefore not surprising that the occurrence of CTS is increased in occupations with manual labor with or without hand-held tools, especially work involving repetitive wrist movements and strenuous work[101-109]. Static work and concomitant ischemia, as when a forcefully flexed or extended posture of the hand and wrist is maintained for a prolonged time, may increase the risk for compression damage to sensitive nerve fibres.[110]

An increased prevalence of CTS has been observed in occupational groups using vibrating tools.[111-116] In an attempt to explain this and the diffuse neuropathy seen in vibration-exposed persons, a pathogenic theory involving vibration as an etiologic factor has been advanced.[117] It is based on the finding in rats that vibration caused epineural edema in the sciatic nerve. Neural edema, by compressing the terminal branches of the median nerve, was also suggested to be responsible for the nocturnal paresthesia seen in some subjects with clinical but not electrodiagnostic signs of CTS. The relevance for humans of these findings is uncertain, for three reasons: (1) it is not obvious that the experimental exposure (vibration at 82 Hz, peak-to-peak amplitude of 0.21 mm) is in any way equivalent to the vibration exposure that may cause disturbances in professional workers; (2) the physiological processes involved in the production of edema in immobilized, anesthetized animals may not be analogous to those occurring in the skin of a person performing dynamic work; (3) support for this theory has not been obtained in epidemiological or physiological studies of vibration-exposed workers or other human subjects.

In general, no epidemiological studies on CTS have been able to make an etiologic distinction, in one and the same occupational group, between vibration and other factors, for instance, repetitive movements and strained wrist postures.

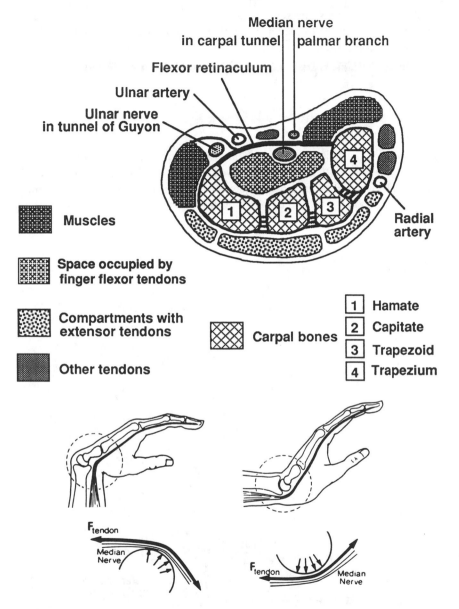

FIGURE 4-8. (Above) the carpal tunnel: distal cutting surface of a transverse section through the wrist. (Below) Pressure on the median nerve in wrist flexion and extension (reproduced with permission from Armstrong and Silverstein 1987[99]).

The *ulnar nerve,* too, passes through a canal at the wrist (Figure 4-9) but is not as strongly susceptible to compression by hand movements and postures. It may, however, become affected by mechanical influence from such factors[118-120] with a consequent sensory deficiency in the corresponding part of the hand.

THE LOCOMOTOR SYSTEM

The bones of the hand-arm system, the joints formed at their contacts, and the muscles attached to them are all involved in work carried out by persons using hand-held vibrating tools. Low-frequency vibration is more readily transmitted along the hand and arm, and this kind of vibration from percussive tools is likely

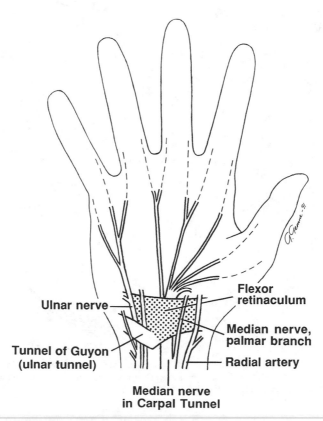

FIGURE 4-9.   The median and ulnar nerves of the wrist.

to reach the wrist and elbow joints in amounts substantial enough to make these organs potential targets.

The epidemiologic documentation of damage to bones and joints in workers exposed to HAV is ambivalent. The specific and nonspecific harmful effects of vibration have been described in a review of the literature by Gemne and Saraste, the pertinent results of which are summarized in the following two sections.[121]

Osteoarthrosis

Investigations performed over several decades on coal miners in the Ruhr area working with hand-held pneumatic tools have demonstrated a slight increase in the risk for osteoarthrosis of the elbow joint.[122, 123] The prevalence attributable to this etiology is low, only about 1 percent. The pathology is said to be produced by percussions from the chipping hammers. Support for this theory comes from animal experiments showing that impact vibration can cause osteoarthrosis[124] by bringing the chondral surfaces into contact with each other. Repeated over a prolonged time, this may damage the cartilage, especially if the joint is held in extreme positions where the cartilage is thinnest. The injury causes disorganization and a subsequent remodeling of the subchondral trabecular bone, which makes the joint surface irregular. These alterations eventually show up in radiograms as a sign of osteoarthrosis.

This increase in the risk for osteoarthrosis, however, is not specific to vibration exposure. A constitutional susceptibility may be required to produce the lesion. Joint load associated with all manual labor, especially when the work is performed in strenuous postures,[125] may result in osteoarthrosis. Joint degeneration may also result when the cartilage is deprived of nutritional substances. Such a situation arises in static work, where a position of the hand and arm is kept for a prolonged time with maintained muscle contraction. This impedes the blood flow to the subarticular bone, from which the cartilage is nourished by diffusion.

Vibration from percussive tools may contribute in yet other ways to an increase of joint load. The contraction that automatically occurs in a muscle exposed to vibration, the tonic vibration reflex,[126] may increase the joint load to some degree.[127] Finally, a percussive tool will wander and jump if it is not handled firmly. To make the tool perform optimally in conjunction with the work piece, the hand joints must be stabilized by a stronger contraction of both flexor and extensor muscles than would be necessary with a nonvibrating tool. The different mechanisms that may induce osteoarthrosis are summarized in Figure 4-10.

Bone Changes

Cysts or vacuoles have often been said to be produced by vibration exposure, but there is no convincing evidence for this in epidemiologic studies. In a radiographic

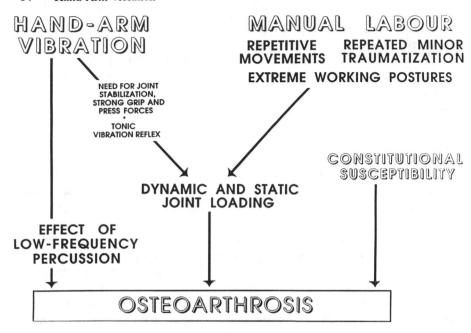

FIGURE 4-10.   Possible mechanisms of osteoarthrosis in manual labor.

examination, by independent radiologists who were unaware of the occupational history of the subjects, Taylor et al.[128] could find no statistically significant difference in bone cyst prevalence between workers engaged in chipping and grinding and manual workers without vibration exposure. A radiological study of chain-sawyers, grinders, and controls without vibration exposure[129] indicated that heavy manual labor may be an important factor in cyst formation.

Kienböck postulated in 1910 that degeneration of the lunate bone in the wrist could arise from trauma, including vibration.[130] The pathogenesis of Kienböck's disease is still incompletely understood (see Chapter 3). The greatest shear on the lunate is when this bone is forced into ulnar deviation. Rossak postulated[131] that this increased stress caused microscopic stress fractures in the lunate. Lee[132] and Kashiwagi et al.[133] have also found microfractures in patients with Kienböck's disease. The role of vibration per se has not yet been validated.

Muscle Function
A reduction of muscular power (hand-grip strength) has been related to vibration exposure.[134, 135] In a two-year follow-up of Finnish forestry workers[136] the loss of muscle force during the two years was 21 percent among subjects with VWF as compared with 5 percent among those without hand-arm symptoms, all with equal vibration exposure. It was stated that this decrease was greater than could be

accounted for by aging. Another observation, however, was that the lumberjacks with a previous history of diminished grip force had actually gained in force by 4 percent. Some other studies have failed to demonstrate reduction in hand-grip force, for instance that of Hellström and Lange Andersen (1972) in forestry workers.[137]

Muscle weakness or dystrophy has been based only on subjective statements, or on current measurements without access to data for the same individuals prior to the beginning of vibration exposure. Muscle exercise commonly leads to a build-up of muscle strength and volume. The possibility that an increase in strength and volume from exercise, and a decrease induced by vibration exposure occur simultaneously in the muscle indicates the difficulties involved in epidemiological studies. No convincing pathogenic mechanisms have yet been documented, although it has been suggested that muscle atrophy and loss of strength may be secondary to motor nerve injury.[138, 139] Prospective investigations, with physiological and histopathological studies are needed to arrive at conclusive evidence in this matter.

DAMAGE TO THE CENTRAL NERVOUS SYSTEM

Vibration Disease—a Soviet Systemic Disorder

In the Soviet Union, Andreeva-Galanina and her co-workers[140-143] developed a classification system for what they called "vibration disease." It was founded on the theory that HAV has a primary effect on the CNS, causing a systemic disorder, which secondarily results in a wide range of symptoms. This classification identified various syndromes: angiodystonic and angiospastic (peripheral circulatory disturbances); vegetative-polyneuritic, myofascitic and neuritic (sensory and motor disturbances, including for instance CTS); diencephalic (diencephalitis) and vestibular. The diencephalic syndrome comprised "generalized vascular crises" in cerebral and coronary vessels resulting in neuropsychiatric symptoms.

Japanese Theory of Damage to the CNS

In the 1960s, some Japanese researchers[144-145] adopted the Soviet views, in support of claims from a group of lumberjacks, that serious and permanent injury to the CNS had been induced by vibration from chain-saws. The Soviet classification of vibration disease was duplicated in the first Japanese guidelines (Japanese Ministry of Labor 1975).[147] Matoba and collaborators[148-150] have been the main advocates of this theory. In the Japanese classification, the symptoms corresponding to the diencephalic syndrome were headache, sleep disturbances, forgetfulness, fatiguability, and impotence.

Pathophysiology and Documentation of "Vibration Disease"

A scrutiny of Soviet literature[150-152] has shown that a validation of the "vibration disease" theory is lacking. There is no evidence that the vibration-induced disorders form a nosologic entity. In Japanese literature, no documentation of damage to central nervous structures have been presented. Neuropsychiatric symptoms seem to have been virtually nonexistent outside Japan, the former Soviet Union and East-European countries. Thus, for instance, Taylor[153] examined 78 advanced HAVS cases but found no disturbances related to the function of the brain or the endocrine system. In Japan, a new classification for clinical use has been recently adopted.[154] It recognizes only the major categories of vibration-induced disturbances used elsewhere comprising disorders in peripheral vascular and neurological functions together with locomotor disturbances. Other disorders are explicitly excluded. The allegations that vibration exposure from hand-held tools had caused neuropsychiatric symptoms have been refuted by the Japanese Supreme Court (Forestry Agency of Japan 1991).[155]

Matoba and his collaborators regarded what they termed vibration disease as induced by the influence on the organism of stressors: noise, cold, and vibration, together with "tension and posture at work." These factors were said to cause an "input overflow" with harmful effects on the limbic system and the cerebral cortex. The subjects developed neuropsychiatric symptoms, such as insomnia, and impotence, as well as tinnitus and hearing loss. Another group of symptoms consisted of secondary disturbances in peripheral, circulatory, and muscular functions. This was believed to occur through the influence of the adrenal medulla and "feedback mechanisms." Another term for this is "defense reaction." The autonomic integration of external and internal stimuli pertinent to these mechanisms has been reviewed by Gemne.[156] There is no reason to question that stressors may have a profound effect on the autonomic nervous system, but the allegation that an "input overflow" can cause chronic or permanent injury (functionally and/or anatomically) has not been validated.

Psychosomatic Reactions to Stressors

The neuropsychiatric symptoms may be regarded as psychosomatic reactions to stress factors, which are well known to occur in susceptible individuals. The working environment of vibration-exposed persons always contains several stressors: vibration, noise, cold, heavy physical work with loading of joints and muscles, and psychological factors such as dissatisfaction with working conditions and salary. Stress factors are also present in the nonoccupational environmental. A conference in London addressed the possible effects of HAV on the central autonomic nervous system. The psychosomatic interpretation was expressed as a collective opinion of the párticipating physicians[157] with the exception of the Japanese proponents of the CNS theory. This is consistent with sound scientific practice. An interpretation based on accepted mechanisms and widespread clinical experience should take precedence over speculative theory.

SUMMARY

The potential target organ systems of vibration from hand-held tools are the finger skin vasculature, sensory nerve structures of the hand, and parts of the locomotor apparatus of the hand-arm system. Available evidence supports the view that HAV syndrome comprises disturbances in these three systems that are pathogenically independent of each other.

The pathogenic events leading to VWF are still unexplained. An increased sympathetic activity may play a role in the development as well as in the manifestation of the disorder. The primary lesion, however, is likely to reside in the skin vessels and their associated vasomotor nerve functions. These functional disturbances may involve endothelial mechanisms and the activity of vasoregulatory receptors or effectors. There are indications of anatomical changes in the vessels such as wall hypertrophy or damage to the endothelium. White finger attacks may involve a cold-induced closure of the digital arteries, but constriction of end vessels in the finger skin also seems necessary. An autonomic imbalance between the sympathetic and parasympathetic nervous systems, induced by vibration exposure and the influence of other stressors, has been suggested to cause a net enhancement of the vasoconstrictory reflex elicited by cold. The relative importance of cold, noise, other physical and psychological stressors, and heavy nicotine consumption in the development of the pathology still eludes us. This is also true for individual factors such as age and the common constitutional tendency to pronounced peripheral vasoconstriction with low skin temperatures in the fingers and toes. It is a physiologically plausible assumption that such a disposition may enhance the susceptibility to harmful vibration. Because of epidemiological difficulties, this and many other important questions concerning vascular disturbances—especially the possibly pathogenic role of cold—still await validation. The suggested relationship between Raynaud's phenomenon and hearing loss in vibration-exposed workers is as yet unclear.

The mechanism for the development of the diffuse neuropathy with sensory deficiency seen in many vibration-exposed workers remains obscure. Mechanical influence from vibration exposure possibly plays a major etiologic role in this disorder, but other ergonomic factors may contribute. The major pathogenic mechanism of carpal tunnel syndrome (CTS) appears to be mechanical insult and compression of the nerve from repetitive, forceful wrist flexion and extension. Excessive flexor tendon use may produce synovitis and swelling with secondary nerve compression, and an increase in intratunnel pressure may result from maintained space-limiting postures of the wrist. An increased prevalence of CTS has been observed in occupational groups using vibrating tools. A pathogenic theory, based on vibration-induced epineural edema in rats, has been advanced to explain CTS and diffuse neuropathy in those workers, but the relevance of the animal data for humans is uncertain. There are no epidemiological studies where an etiologic distinction has been made between vibration and other factors, for instance repetitive, forceful movements and strained wrist postures. The ulnar nerve at the wrist, although less susceptible, may become mechanically affected by ergonomic factors, with a consequent sensory deficiency in the corresponding part of the hand.

The chief etiologic factor behind wrist and elbow osteoarthrosis observed at a low prevalence in some vibration-exposed workers is probably the load associated with heavy manual work, but a constitutional susceptibility may be required. A contribution to osteoarthrosis may come from repeated shocks to the chondral surfaces caused by percussions, particularly in extreme postures of the joints, and the extra load associated with manipulating of a vibrating tool. The role of vibration for anatomical changes in bones and for a possible reduction in muscle power is still unclarified.

In addition to peripheral vascular disturbances, damage to the central nervous system by HAV has been alleged to cause neuropsychiatric symptoms and chronic changes in the autonomic regulation of organ systems such as the heart. The pathophysiology of this theory has not been clarified. Symptoms occurring outside the hand and arm in vibration-exposed persons reflect an unspecific autonomic dysfunction and are indistinguishable from psychosomatic manifestations of environmental physical and psychological stressors.

Notes

1. Gemne, G., ed. Stockholm Workshop 86. "Symptomatology and Diagnostic Methods in the Hand-Arm Vibration Syndrome." *Scand. J. Work Environ. Health* 1987; 13 (4 Spec. issue): 265–388.
2. Olsen, N. "Vibration-Induced white finger. Physiological and Clinical Aspects" (Thesis). Copenhagen: Laegeforeningens Forlag. 1988.
3. Olsen, N. "Hyperreactivity of the Central Sympathetic Nervous System in Vibration-Induced White Finger". *Kurume Med. J.* 1990; 37(Suppl): S109–S116.
4. Olsen, "Vibration-Induced White Finger."
5. Färkkilä, M.; Pyykkö, I.; Heinonen, E. "Vibration Stress and the Autonomic Nervous System." *Kurume Med. J.* 1990; 37 (Suppl): S53–S60.
6. Bannister, R. "Chronic Autonomic Failure With Postural Hypotension." *The Lancet* 1979; i: 404–406.
7. Bruyn, G. W. "Vibration-Induced Central Dysautonomia. Fact or Fiction?" In: Gemne, G.; Taylor, W., eds. *Hand-Arm Vibration and the Central Autonomic Nervous System*. Proc. Intern. Symp., London 1983. *J Low Freq. Noise Vibr.* 1983; (1 Spec. Issue): 100–107.

8. Bovenzi, M. "Autonomic Stimulation and Cardiovascular Reflex Activity in the Hand-Arm Vibration Syndrome." *Kurume Med. J.* 1990; 37:S85–S94.

9. Heinonen, E.; Färkkilä, M.; Forsström, J.; Antila, K.; Jalonen, J.; Korhonen, O.; Pyykkö, I., "Autonomic Neuropathy and Vibration Exposure in Forestry Workers." *Br. J. Ind. Med.* 1987; 44:412–416.

10. Harada, N.; Nakamoto, M.; Kohno, H.; Kondo, H.; Tanaka, M. "Hormonal Responses to Cold Exposure in Subjects With Vibration Syndrome." *Kurume Med. J.* 1990; 37 (Suppl): S45–S52.

11. Spittell, Jr, J. A. "Raynaud's Phenomenon and Allied Vasospastic Conditions." In: Fairbairn J. F.; Juergens, J. L.; Spittell, Jr, J. A.; eds. *Peripheral Vascular Diseases. 4th ed.* Philadelphia: WB Saunders Co, 1972: 387–419.

12. Leppert, J. "Primary Raynaud's Phenomenon in Women" (Thesis). Acta Univ. Upsal. No. 223, Stockholm: Almqvist & Wiksell International, 1989.

13. Nielsen, S. L.; Sörensen, C.; Olsen, N. "Thermostated Measurement of Systolic Blood Pressure on Cooled Finger." *Scand. J. Clin. Invest.* 1980; 40:683–687.

14. Corbin, D. O. C.; Wood, D. A.; Housley, E. "An Evaluation of Finger Systolic-Pressure Response to Local Cooling in the Diagnosis of Primary Raynaud's phenomenon." *Clin. Physiol.* 1985; 5:383–392.

15. Coffman, J. D., and Cohen, A. S. "Total and Capillary Blood Flow in Raynaud's Phenomenon." *New Engl. J. Med.* 1971; 285:259–263.

16. Downey, J. A., and Frewin, D. B. "The Effect of Cold on Blood Flow in the Hands of Patients With Raynaud's Phenomenon". *Clin. Sci.* 1973; 44: 279.

17. Fagius, J.; and Blumberg, H. "Sympathetic Outflow to the Hand in Patients With Raynaud's Phenomenon". *Cardiovasc. Res.* 1985; 19:249.

18. Kontos, H. A. and Wasserman, A. J. "Effect of Reserpine in Raynaud's Phenomenon." *Circulation* 1969; 39:259.

19. Lewis, T. "Observations Upon the Reactions of the Vessels of the Human Skin to Cold." *Heart* 1930; 15:177–208.

20. Leppert, "Primary Raynaud's Phenomenon in Women."

21. Kahan, A.; Weber, S.; Amor, B.; Menkes, C. J.; Saporta, L.; Hodara, M.; Guerin, F.; Degeorges, M. "Calcium Entry Blocking Agents in Digital Vasospasm (Raynaud's Phenomenon)." *Eur. Heart. J.* 1983; 4(Suppl. C): 123–129.

22. Linder, H. R.; Reinhart, W.; Mahler, F. "Local Cooling Test (LCT) for Provocation of Nailfold Capillary Flow Changes in Vasospastic and Rheological Disorders." Abstr. 5th World Congress for Microcirculation. Louisville, Kentucky, Sept. 1991:62.

23. Martini, R.; Di Pino, L.; Monaco, S.; Palazzo, V.; Signorelli, S.; Andreozzi, G. M. "The Prevalence of a Cyanotic Phase in Raynaud's Phenomenon." Abstr. 5th World Congress for Microcirculation. Louisville, Kentucky. Sept. 1991:69.

24. Gemne, G.; Pyykkö, I.; Taylor, W.; Pelmear, P. L. "The Stockholm Workshop Scale for the Classification of Cold-Induced Raynaud's Phenomenon in the Hand-Arm Vibration Syndrome (Revision of the Taylor-Pelmear Scale). *Scand. J. Work. Environ. Health.* 1987; 13 (Special issue 4): 275–278.

25. Nielsen, S. L. and Lassen, N. A. "Measurement of Digital Blood Pressure After Local Cooling." *J. Appl. Physiol.* 1977; 43:907–910.

26. Olsen, N. and Nielsen, S. L. "Diagnosis of Raynaud's Phenomenon in Quarrymen's Traumatic Vasospastic Disease." *Scand. J. Work. Environ. Health* 1979; 5:249–256.

27. Furchgott, R. "Role of the Endothelium in Response of Vascular Smooth Muscle." *Circ. Res.* 1983; 53:557–573.
28. Endrich, B. "Microvascular Ultrastructure in Non-Freezing Cold Injuries. A Clinical Model to Study Reperfusion Injury?" Abstr. 5th World Congress for Microcirculation. Louisville, Kentucky, Sept. 1991:24.
29. Jamieson, G. G.; Ludbrook, J.; Wilson, A. "Cold Hypersensitivity in Raynaud's Phenomenon." *Circulation* 1971; 44:254–64.
30. Ekenvall, L. and Lindblad, L. E. "Is Vibration White Finger a Primary Sympathetic Injury?" *Br. J. Ind. Med* 1986; 43:702–706.
31. Vanhoutte, P. P.; Cooke, J. P.; Lindblad L. E.; Shepherd, J. T.; Flavahan, N. A. "Modulation of Postjunctional Alpha-Adrenergic Responsiveness by Local Changes in Temperature." *Clin. Sci.* 1985; 68:121–135.
32. Flavahan, N. A.; Lindblad, L. E.; Verbeuren, T. J.; Shepherd, J. T.; Vanhoutte, P. M. Cooling and Alpha$_1$ and Alpha$_2$-Adrenergic Responses in Cutaneous Veins: Role of Receptor Reserve." *Am. J. Physiol.* 1985; 249: H950–H955.
33. Ekenvall, L.; Lindblad, L. E.; Norbeck, O.; Etzell, B. M. "Alpha-Adrenoceptors and Cold-Induced Vasoconstriction in Human Finger Skin." *Am. J. Physiol.* 1988; 255:H1000–H1003.
34. Lindblad, L. E.; and Ekenvall, L. "Alpha$_2$-Adrenoceptor Inhibition in Patients With Vibration White Fingers." *Kurume Med. J.* 1990; 37 (Suppl): S95–S99.
35. Bodelsson, M.; Arneklo-Nobin, B.; Nobin, A.; Owman, C; Sollerman, C.; Törnebrandt, K. "Cooling Enhances Alpha$_2$-Adrenoceptor Mediated Vasoconstriction in Human Hand Veins." *Acta. Physiol. Scand.* 1990; 138:283–291.
36. Zelis, R. "Mechanisms of Vasodilation." *Am. J. Med.* June 27, 1983: 3–12.
37. Bodelsson, M.; Arneklo-Nobin, B.; Törnebrandt, K. "Effect of Cooling on Smooth Muscle Response to 5-Hydroxytryptamine in Human Hand Veins." *Acta Physiol Scand.* 1990; 140:331–339.
38. Bodelsson, M. "Vascular Effects of Cooling. With Special References to Human Serotonergic, Adrenergic, and Endothelial Mechanisms" (Thesis). Bulletin No. 77, Department of Surgery. Lund University, 1990.
39. Schwinn, D.; Caron, M.; Lefkowitz, R. J. "Molecular Biology of Adrenoceptors." Abstr. 5th World Congress for Microcirculation. Louisville, Kentucky, Sept. 1991:99.
40. Bradley, P. B.; Engel, G.; Feniuk, W.; Fozard, J. R.; Humphrey, P. P. A.; Middlemiss, D. N.; Mylecharane, E. J.; Richardson, B. P.; Saxena, P. R. Proposals for the Classification and Nomenclature of Functional Receptors for 5-Hydroxytryptamine. *Neuropharmacology.* 1986; 25:563–576.
41. Gemne, G.; Pyykkö, I.; Inaba, R. "Finger Blood Flow Reaction to Iontophoresis of Metacholine and Nitroprusside in Chain-Sawyers With and Without White Fingers." In: Abstr. 6th Int Conf. of Hand-Arm Vibration, Bonn, Germany, May 1992, pp. 23–24.
42. Moulds R. F. W.; Iwanov, V.; Medcalf, R. L. "The Effect of Platelet-Derived Contractile Agents on Human Digital Arteries." *Clin. Sci.* 1984; 66:443–451.
43. Pyykkö, I.; Gemne, G.; Kolari, P.; Starck, J.; Ilmarinen, R.; Aalto, H. "Vasomotor Oscillation in Vibration-Induced White Finger." *Scand. J. Work. Environ. Health* 1986; 12 (4 Spec. issue): 395–399.
44. Hyvärinen, J.; Pyykkö, I.; Sundberg, S. "Vibration Frequencies and Amplitudes in the Etiology of Traumatic Vasospastic Disease." *The Lancet* 1973; i:791–794.

45. Gemne, G. "Pathophysiology and Multifactorial Etiology of Acquired Vasospastic Disease (Raynaud Syndrome) in Vibration-Exposed Workers." *Scand. J. Work. Environ. Health* 1982; 8:243-249.
46. Ibid.
47. Walton, K. W. "The Pathology of Raynaud's Phenomenon of Occupational Origin." In: Taylor, W., ed. *The Vibration Syndrome.* London: Academic Press, 1974:109-119.
48. Takeuchi, T.; Futatsuka, M.; Imanishi, H. "Pathological Changes Observed in the Finger Biopsy of Patients With Vibration-Induced White Finger." *Scand. J. Work. Environ. Health* 1986; 12(4 Spec. issue): 280-283.
49. Takeuchi, T. and Imanishi, H. "Histopathologic Observations in Finger Biopsy From Thirty Patients With Raynaud's Phenomenon of Occupational Origin." *J. Kumamoto Med. Soc.* 1984; 58:56-70.
50. Okada, A. "Pathogenic Mechanisms of Vibration-Induced White Finger (VWF)—Recent Findings and Speculations." In: Okada, A.; Taylor, W.; Dupuis, H.; eds. *Hand-Arm Vibration.* Kanazawa, Japan: Kyoei Press Co., 1990:1-8.
51. Ross, R.; Glomet, J.; Harker, L. "Response to Injury and Atherogenesis. *Amer. J. Pathol.* 1977; 86:675-684.
52. Okada, A.; Inaba, R.; Furuno, T.; Nohara, S.; Ariizumi, M. "Usefulness of Blood Parameters, Especially Viscosity, for the Diagnosis and Elucidation of Pathogenic Mechanisms of the Hand-Arm Vibration Syndrome." *Scand. J. Work. Environ. Health* 1987; 13(4 Spec. issue): 358-362.
53. Okada, "Pathogenic Mechanisms."
54. Guyton, A. C. *Textbook of Medical Physiology. 7th ed.* Philadelphia: WB Saunders Co, 1986:1057.
55. Gemne, G.; Pyykkö, I.; Starck, J.; Ilmarinen, R. "Circulatory Reaction to Heat and Cold in Vibration-Induced White Finger with and without Sympathetic Blockade. An Experimental Study." Scand. J. Work Environ. Health 1986 (4 Spec. issue): 371-377.
56. Ibid.
57. Pyykkö, I.; Kolari, P.; Färkkilä, M.; Starck, J.; Korhonen, O.; Jäntti, V. "Finger Peripheral Resistance During Local Cold Provocation in Vasospastic Disease." *Scand. J. Work. Environ. Health* 1986; 12(4 Spec. issue): 395-399.
58. Wegelius, U. "Angiography of the hand. Clinical and postmortem investigations" (Thesis). *Acta Radiol.* 1972; Suppl. 315:1-115.
59. Arneklo-Nobin, B. "The Objective Diagnosis of Vibration-Induced Vascular Injury." *Scand. J. Work. Environ. Health* 1987; 13(4 Spec. issue): 337-342.
60. Gemne, "Pathophysiology and Multifactorial Etiology."
61. Ibid.
62. Bodelsson, Arneklo-Noblin, and Törnebrandt, "Effect of Cooling."
63. Lundborg, G.; Dahlin, L. B.; Danielsen, N.; Hansson, H. A.; Necking, L. E. "Intraneural Edema Following Exposure to Vibration." *Scand. J. Work. Environ. Health* 1987; 13 (4 Spec. issue): 326-329.
64. Hayward, R. A. and Griffin, M. J. "Hand-Transmitted Vibration, Vibrotactile Thresholds and Vibration-Induced White Finger." (Awaiting publication; quoted in Griffin, M. J. *Handbook of Human Vibration.* Academic Press, London 1990: 601)

65. Pyykkö, I.; Starck, J.; Färkkilä, M.; Hoikkala, M.; Korhonen, O.; Nurminen, M. "Hand-Arm Vibration in the Etiology of Hearing Loss in Lumberjacks. *Br. J. Ind. Med.* 1981; 38:281-289.

66. Pyykkö, I. and Starck, J. "Vibration Syndrome in the Etiology of Occupational Hearing Loss." *Acta Otolaryngol.* (Stockholm) 1982; 386(Suppl.): 296-300.

67. Iki, M.; Kurumatani, N.; Moriyama, T. "Vibration-Induced White Fingers and Hearing Loss." *The Lancet* 1983; ii:282-283.

68. Iki, M.; Kurumatani, N.; Hirata, K.; Moriyama, T. "An Association Between Raynaud's Phenomenon and Hearing Loss in Forestry Workers." *Amer. Ind. Hyg. Assoc. J.* 1985; 46:509-513.

69. Iki, M.; Kurumatani, N.; Hirata, K.; Moriyama, T.; Satoh, M.; Arai, T. "Association Between Vibration-Induced White Finger and Hearing Loss in Forestry Workers." *Scand. J. Work. Environ. Health* 1986; 12:365-370.

70. Iki, M.; Kurumatani, N.; Satoh, M.; Matsuura, F.; Arai, T.; Ogata, A.; Moriyama, T. "Hearing of Forest Workers with Vibration-Induced White Finger: A Five-Year Follow-up." *Int. Arch. Occup. Environ. Health* 1989; 61:437-442.

71. Miyakita, T.; Miura, H.; Futatsuka, M. "Noise-Induced Hearing Loss in Relation to Vibration-Induced White Finger in Chain Saw Workers." *Scand. J. Work. Environ. Health* 1987; 13:32-36.

72. Pelmear, P. L.; Leong, D.; Wong, L.; Roos, J.; Pike, M. "Hand-Arm Vibration Syndrome and Hearing Loss in Hard Rock Miners." *J. Low Freq. Noise Vib.* 1987; 6(2):49-66.

73. Pyykkö, I.; Pekkarinen, J.; Starck, J. "Sensory-Neural Hearing Loss During Combined Noise and Vibration Exposure." *Int. Arch. Occup. Environ. Health* 1987; 59:439-454.

74. Pyykkö, I.; Starck, J.; Pekkarinen, J. "Further Evidence of a Relation Between Noise-Induced Permanent Threshold Shift and Vibration-Induced Digital Vasospasms." *Am. J. Otolaryngol.* 1986; 4:391-398.

75. Pyykkö, I.; Koskimies, K.; Starck, J.; Pekkarinen, J.; Färkkilä, M.; Inaba, R. "Risk Factors in the Genesis of Sensorineural Hearing Loss in Finnish Forestry Workers." *Br. J. Ind. Med.* 1989; 46:439-446.

76. Iki, M.; Kuramatani, N.; Moriyama, T.; Ogata, A. "Vibration-Induced White Finger and Auditory Susceptibility to Noise Exposure." *Kurume Med. J.* 1990; 37:33-34.

77. Starck, J.; Pekkarinen, J.; Pyykkö, I. "Impulse Noise and Hand-Arm Vibration in Relation to Sensory Neural Hearing Loss." *Scand. J. Work. Environ. Health* 1988; 14:265-271.

78. Starck, J.; Pekkarinen, J.; Liu, Chang Chun. "Transmission of Vibration From Tool Handle to Wrist and Head." *Kurume Med. J.* 1990; 37(Suppl.): S1-S11.

79. Arikawa, K.; Shirakawa, T.; Kotorii, T.; Oshima, M.; Nakazawa, Y.; Inanaga, K.; Kuwahara, K. "An Electroencephalographic Study of Patients With Vibration Disease." *Folia Psychiat. Neurol. Jap.* 1978; 32:211-222.

80. Koishizawa, M.; Inami, Y.; Inoda, Y.; Inoue, K.; Horio, K.; Kamihara, M. "EEG Findings in Patients With Vibration Syndrome." In: Okada, A.; Taylor, W.; Dupuis, H., eds. *Hand-Arm Vibration.* Kanazawa, Japan: Kyoei Press Co., 1990:279-282.

81. Harada, N.; Kondo, H.; Kohno, H.; Nakamoto, M.; Yoshida, I.; Kimura, K. "Investigations of Autonomic Nervous Function in Vibration Syndrome Using Heart Rate Variation, Serum Dopamine-Betahydroxylase and Plasma Cyclic Nucleotides." In:

Okada, A.; Taylor, W.; Dupuis, H., eds. *Hand-Arm Vibration*. Kanazawa, Japan: Kyoei Press Co., 1990: 267-272.

82. Harada, Nakamoto, Kohno, Kondo, and Tanaka, "Hormonal Responses."
83. Ibid.
84. Ekenvall, L. and Lindblad, L. E. "Effect of Tobacco Use on Vibration White Finger Disease." *J. Occup. Med.* 1989; 30(1): 13-16.
85. Virokannas, H.; Anttonen, H.; Pramila, S. "Combined Effect of Hand-Arm Vibration and Smoking on White Finger in Different Age Groups." *Archives of Complex Environmental Studies* 1991; 3(1-2):7-12.
86. Pyykkö, I. "The Prevalence and Symptoms of Traumatic Vasospastic Disease Among Lumberjacks in Finland. A Field Study." *Work-environm-hlth* 1974; 11:118-131.
87. Pelnar, P. V.; Gibbs, G. W.; Pathak, B. P. "A Pilot Investigation of the Vibration Syndrome in Forestry Workers of Eastern Canada." In: Brammer, A. J. and Taylor, W., eds. *Vibration Effects on the Hand and Arm in Industry*. New York: John Wiley & Sons, 1982:173-187.
88. Nilsson, T.; Burström, L.; Hagberg, M. "Risk Assessment of Vibration Exposure and White Fingers Among Platers." *Int. Arch. Occup. Environ. Health* 1989; 61:473-481.
89. Färkkilä, M. and Pyykkö, I. "Blood Flow in the Contralateral Hand During Vibration and Hand Grip Contractions of Lumberjacks." *Scand. J. Work. Environ. Health* 1979; 5:368-370.
90. Pyykkö, I. and Hyvärinen, J. "The Physiological Basis of the Traumatic Vasospastic Disease: A Sympathetic Vasoconstrictor Reflex Triggered by High Frequency Vibration? *Work-environm. hlth* 1973; 10:36-47.
91. Skoglund, C. R. and Knutsson, E. "Vasomotor Changes in Human Skin Elicited by High Frequency Low Amplitude Vibration." *Acta Physiol. Scand.* 1985; 125:335-336.
92. Skoglund, C. R. "Vasodilatation in Human Skin Induced by Low-Amplitude High Frequency Vibration." *Clin. Physiol.* 1989; 9:361-372.
93. Ljung, N. and Sivertsson, R. "Vibration-Induced Inhibition of Vascular Smooth Muscle Contraction." *Blood Vessels* 1975; 12:38-52.
94. Lundborg, Dahlin, Danielsen, Hansson, and Necking, "Intraneural Edema."
95. Takeuchi, T.; Futatsuka, M.; Imanishi, H.; Yamada, S. "Pathological Changes Observed in the Finger Biopsy of Patients with Vibration-Induced White Finger." *Scand. J. Work Environ. Health 1986*; 12:280-283.
96. Ekenvall, L.; Nilsson, B. Y.; Gustavsson, P. "Temperature and Vibration Thresholds in Vibration Syndrome." *Br. J. Ind. Med.* 1986; 43:825-829.
97. Ekenvall, L.; Nilsson, B. Y.; Falconer, C. "Sensory Perception in the Hands of Dentists." *Scand. J. Work. Environ. Health* 1990; 16:334-339.
98. Brezinova, V. and Quinton, D. N. "Response to Cold and Abnormalities of Nerve Conduction Velocity in Hand-Arm Vibration Syndrome." *Br. J. Ind. Med.* 1991; 48:353-354.
99. Armstrong, T. J., and Silverstein, B. A., "Upper-extremity pain in the workplace. Role of usage in causality" In: Hadler, N. M. ed. "Clinical Concepts in Regional Musculo-skeletal Illness", New York: Grune & Stratton, Inc. 1987, pp. 333-354.

100. Armstrong, T. J.; Castelli, W. A.; Evans, F. G.; Diaz-Perez, R. "Some Histological Changes in Carpal Tunnel Contents and their Biomechanical Implication." *J. Occup. Med.* 1984; 26:197–201.
101. Ahlborg, Jr., G. and Voog, L. "Vibration Exposure and Distal Compression of the Median Nerve (Carpal Tunnel Syndrome)." *Läkartidningen (J. Swedish Med. Assoc.)* 1982; 79:4905–4908.
102. Cannon, L. J.; Bernacki, E. J.; Walther, S. D. "Personal and Occupational Factors Associated With Carpal Tunnel Syndrome." *J. Occup. Med.* 1981; 23:255–258.
103. Armstrong, T. J.; Fine, L. J.; Radwin, R. G.; Silverstein, B. S. "Ergonomics and the Effects of Vibration in Hand-Intensive Work." *Scand. J. Work Environ. Health* 1987 (4 Spec. issue):286–289.
104. Carragee, E. J., and Hentz, R. "Repetitive Trauma and Nerve Compression." *Orthop. Clin. North Am.* 1988; 19:157–164.
105. Falck, B. and Aarnio, P. "Left-Sided Carpal Tunnel Syndrome in Butchers." *Scand. J. Work. Environ. Health* 1983; 9:291–297.
106. Margolis, W. and Kraus, J. F. "The Prevalence of Carpal Tunnel Syndrome Symptoms in Female Supermarket Checkers." *J. Occup. Med.* 1987; 29:953–956.
107. Silverstein, B. A.; Fine, L. J.; Armstrong, T. J. "Occupational Factors and Carpal Tunnel Syndrome." *Am. J. Ind. Med.* 1987; 11:343–358.
108. Wieslander, G.; Norbäck, D.; Göthe, C.-J.; Juhlin, L. "Carpal Tunnel Syndrome (CTS) and Exposure to Vibration, Repetitive Wrist Movements, and Heavy Manual Work: A Case-Referent Study." *Br. J. Ind. Med.* 1989; 46:43–47.
109. Barnhart, S.; Demers, P. A.; Miller, M.; Longstreth Jr, W. T.; Rosenstock, L. "Carpal Tunnel Syndrome Among Ski Manufacturing Workers." *Scand. J. Work. Environ. Health* 1991; 17:46–52.
110. Gelberman, R. H.; Rydevik, B. L.; Pess, G. M.; Szabo, R. M.; Lundborg, G. "Carpal Tunnel Syndrome." A Scientific Basis for Clinical Care." *Orthop. Clin. North Am.* 1988; 19:115–124.
111. Cannon et al., "Personal and Occupational Factors."
112. Ahlborg and Voog, "Vibration Exposure."
113. Chatterjee, D. S.; Barwick, D. D.; Petrie, A. "Exploratory Electromyography in the Study of Vibration-Induced White Finger in Rock Drillers." *Br. J. Ind. Med.* 1982; 39:89–97.
114. Wieslander, Norbäck, Göthe, Juhlin, "Carpal Tunnel Syndrome."
115. Färkkilä, M.; Koskimies, K.; Pyykkö, I.; Jäntti, V.; Starck, J.; Aatola, S.; Korhonen, O. "Carpal Tunnel Syndrome Among Forest Workers." In: Okada, A.; Taylor, W.; Dupuis, H.; eds. *Hand-Arm Vibration.* Kanazawa, Japan: Kyoei Press Co. 1990:263–265.
116. Nilsson, T.; Hagberg, M.; Burström, L.; Lundström, R. "Prevalence and Odds Ratios of Numbness and Carpal Tunnel Syndrome in Different Exposure Categories of Platers." In: Okada, A.; Taylor, W.; Dupuis, H.; eds. *Hand-Arm Vibration.* Kanazawa, Japan: Kyoei Press Co. 1990:235–239.
117. Lundborg, Dahlin, Danielson, Hansson, Necking, "Intraneural Edema."
118. Eckman, P. B.; Perlstein, G.; Altrocchi, P. H. "Ulnar Neuropathy in Bicycle Riders." *Arch. Neurol.* 1975; 32:130–131.
119. Dupont, C.; Cloutier, G. E.; Prevost, Y., et al. "Ulnar Tunnel Syndrome at the Wrist." *J. Bone Joint Surg.* 1965; 47A: 757–761.

120. Mosely, L. H.; Kalafut, R. M.; Levinson, P. D.; Mokris, S. A. "Cumulative Trauma Disorders and Compression Neuropathies of the Upper Extremities." In: Kasdan, M. L., ed. *Occupational Hand & Upper Extremity Injuries & Diseases.* Philadelphia: Hanley & Belfus, Inc. 1991, pp. 353–402.

121. Gemne, G. and Saraste, H. "Bone and Joint Pathology in Workers Using Hand-Held Vibrating Tools." *Scand. J. Work. Environ. Health* 1987; 13(4 Spec. issue): 290–300.

122. Laarmann, A. "Berufskrankheiten nach mechanischen Einwirkungen." Stuttgart: Enke Verlag, 1977.

123. Rehm, S. "Chronische Wirkungen auf das Knochenund Gelenksystem." In: Dupuis, H., ed. *Wirkung mechanischer Schwingungen auf das Hand-Arm-System.* Expertenkolloquium 1982. Forschungsbericht 348. Bundesanstalt für Arbeitsschutz und Unfallsforschung. Dortmund 1983; 19–28.

124. Radin, E. L.; Parker, H.; Pugh, J.; Steinberg, R.; Paul, I.; Rose, R. "Response of Joints to Impact Loading: III. Relationship Between Trabecular Microfractures and Cartilage Degeneration." *J. Biomech.* 1973; 6:51–57.

125. Anderson, J. A. "Arthrosis and Its Relation to Work." *Scand. J. Work. Environ. Health* 1984; 10:429–433.

126. Hagbarth, K. E. and Eklund, G. "Motor Effects of Vibratory Muscle Stimuli in Man." In: Granit, R., ed. *Muscular Afferents and Motor Control.* New York: John Wiley & Sons, 1965; 177–186.

127. Radwin, R. G.; Armstrong, T. J.; Chaffin, D. B. "Power Hand Tool Vibration Effects on Grip Exertions." *Ergonomics* 1987; 30(5): 833–855.

128. Taylor, W.; Howie, G.; Rappaport, M. "Vibration Syndrome in Chipping and Grinding Workers." *J. Occup. Med.* 1984; 26:765–778.

129. James, P. B.; Yates, J. R.; Pearson, J. C. G. "An Investigation of the Prevalence of Bone Cysts in Hands Exposed to Vibration." In: Taylor, W. and Pelmear, P. L., eds. *Vibration White Finger in Industry.* London: Academic Press, 1975:43–52.

130. Stahl, S. and Reis, N. D. "Traumatic Ulnar Variance in Kienbock's Disease." *J. Hand Surg.* 1986; 11A (1): 95–97.

131. Rossak, K. "Druckverhaltnisse am Handgelenk unter besonderer Berücksichtigung von Fraktur-Mechanismen." *Z. Orthop.* 1967; 103 (Suppl.): 296–299.

132. Lee, M. "The Intraosseous Arterial Pattern of the Carpal Lunate Bone and Its Relation to Avascular Necrosis." *Acta Orthop. Scand.* 1963; 33:43–55.

133. Kashiwagi, D.; Fukiwava, A.; Inone, T.; Liang, F. H.; Imamoto, Y. "An Experimental and Clinical Study on Lunato-Malacia." *Orthop. Trans.* 1977; 1:7.

134. Färkkilä, M. "Grip Force in Vibration Disease." *Scand. J. Work. Environ. Health* 1978; 4:159–166.

135. Färkkilä, M.; Pyykkö, I.; Korhonen, O. "Vibration Induced Decrease in the Muscle Force in Lumberjacks." *Eur. J. Appl. Physiol.* 1980; 43:1–9.

136. Färkkilä, M.; Aatola, S.; Starck, J.; Korhonen, O.; Pyykkö, I. "Hand-Grip Force in Lumberjacks: Two-Year Follow-up." *Int. Arch. Occup. Environ. Health* 1986; 58:203–208.

137. Hellström, B. and Lange Andersen, K. "Vibration Injuries in Norwegian Forest Workers." *Brit. J. Ind. Med.* 1972; 29:255–263.

138. Färkkilä et al. "Hand-Grip Force."

139. Färkkilä, M. "Vibration Induced Injury." *Br. J. Ind. Med.* 1986; 43:361–362.
140. Andreeva-Galanina, E. T. "La maladie vibratoire, son étiologie, patologoie et prophylaxie." In: *Proc XII. Congr. Occup. Health, ICOH.* Helsinki, 1957:385–386.
141. Drogichina, E. A. and Metlina, N. B. "A Contribution to the Vibration Disease Classification." *Gig. Tr. Prof. Zabol.* 1967; (5): 27–31 (in Russian).
142. Andreeva-Galanina, E. T.; Drogichina, E. A.; Artamonova, V. G. *Vibration Disease.* Leningrad: Medgiz 1961 (in Russian).
143. Gemne, G. "Soviet Documentation of Neuro-Psychiatric Symptoms in the Hand-Arm Vibration Syndrome." In: Gemne, G. and Taylor, W., eds. "Hand-Arm Vibration and the Central Autonomic Nervous System." Proc. Intern. Symp. London 1983. *J. Low Freq. Noise Vibr.* 1983; (1 Spec. issue):129–134.
144. Yamada, S. "Vibration Hazards in Japan." *Proc. XVI. Int. Congr. Occup. Health, ICOH,* Tokyo, 1969:139–140.
145. Matoba, T.; Kusumoto, H.; Takamatsu, M. "A New Criterion of the Severity of the Vibration Disease." *Jap. J. Ind. Health* 1975; 17:211–214.
146. Matoba, T.; Kusumoto, H.; Kuwahara, H.; Inanaga, K.; Oshima, M.; Takamatsu, M.; Esaki, K. "Pathophysiology of Vibration Disease." *Jap. J. Ind. Health* 1975; 17:11–18.
147. Japanese Ministry of Labour. Notification No. 608 1975.
148. Matoba, Kusumoto, Takamatsu, "A New Criterion."
149. Matoba, Kusumoto, Kuwahara, Inanaga, Oshima, Takematsu, and Esaki, "Pathophysiology of Vibration Disease."
150. Matoba, T.; Chiba, M., Inutsuka, S. "Autonomic Nervous System Disorders in Subjects Exposed to Hand-Arm Vibration. A Review of Clinical Investigations in Japan." In: Gemne, G. and Taylor, W., eds. *Hand-Arm Vibration and the Central Autonomic Nervous System.* Proc. Intern. Symp., London 1983. *J. Low Freq. Noise Vib.* 1983; (1 Spec issue): 74–83.
151. Gemne, "Soviet Documentation."
152. Gemne, G. " 'Vibration Disease' as a Central Nervous System Disorder. Development, Symptomatology, and Pathophysiology of Soviet and Japanese Classifications." In: Gemne, G., and Taylor, W., eds. "Hand-Arm Vibration and the Central Autonomic Nervous System." Proc. Intern. Symp. London, 1983. *J. Low Freq. Noise Vib.* 1983; (1 Spec. issue): 19–35.
153. Taylor, W.; Ogston, S. A.; Brammer, A. J. "A Clinical Assessment of Seventy-Eight Cases of Hand-Arm Vibration Syndrome." *Scand. J. Work. Environ. Health* 1986; 12(4 Spec. issue): 265–268.
154. Japanese Ministry of Labour, Labour Standards Bureau. Report on Treatment of Vibration Disease, July 1986.
155. Forestry Agency of Japan. A Summary of Hand-Arm Vibration Syndrome Judgments. (Administrative Department. Welfare Division) 1991.
156. Gemne, G. "Autonomic Integration of External and Internal Stimuli, and the Soviet Concept of 'diencephalic syndrome'. " In: Gemne, G., and Taylor, W., eds. "Hand-Arm Vibration and the Central Autonomic Nervous System." Proc. Intern. Symp. London, 1983. *J. Low Freq. Noise Vib.* 1983; (1 Spec. issue): 63–68.
157. Gemne, G., and Taylor, W., eds. "Hand-Arm Vibration and the Central Autonomic Nervous System." Proc. Intern. Symp. London, 1983. *J. Low Freq. Noise Vib.* 1983; (1 Spec. issue): xi.

5

Clinical Evaluation

P. L. Pelmear, W. Taylor

The clinical evaluation of a patient with hand-arm vibration syndrome (HAVS) will vary according to the purpose of the examination and the role of the examining physician, field researcher, worker physician, family physician, or consultant. The subject's history will be very important in any epidemiological study to determine the HAVS prevalence. In these circumstances, the clinical examination may be minimal.[1,2] Time constraints in field studies will limit the depth and quality of the evaluation, so the two essential components must be a questionnaire on the medical and work history and simple clinical tests to confirm the presence of vascular and neurological impairment. Tests to demonstrate the patency of the major vessels, and the response of the digital vessels to immersion in cold water, are feasible and practical, as are neurological tests to determine skin sensitivity to touch, pain, temperature and vibration. Grip strength, as well as hearing loss by audiometry should also be measured. Because the different components of HAVS (for example, finger blanching, numbing of the hands and arms, muscle fatigue) may arise independently, they must be evaluated separately.[3]

When the clinical evaluation is to confirm the diagnosis and to assess the severity of both the vascular and sensorineural stages, the examination has to be extended. The work and medical history must be more detailed and very complete; the physical examination must assess the musculoskeletal, cardiovascular, and neurological systems; and multiple laboratory tests must be used since no single test by itself is diagnostic.[4,5] Several of the tests described in the following pages will have to be used because of the low (50–90 percent) specificity and sensitivity. The selection will depend on the personal preference of the physician and the instrumentation available for screening and for extensive diagnostic evaluation.

77

OCCUPATIONAL AND MEDICAL HISTORY

A complete history of the presenting symptoms (frequency and extent of finger blanching, numbness, tingling), past and present medical history, family history, and occupational history with emphasis on the nature and length of past and present exposure to vibratory tools are essential. An example of a questionnaire that may be used as a checklist guide for field surveys or clinical evaluation in the consulting room or hospital is given in Appendix 1.

The medical history should specifically elicit any history of hand-arm trauma and symptoms to exclude other causes of finger blanching and neurological disorders (for example, possible collagen or rheumatoid disease, large blood vessel obstruction, hematological dyscrasias, and the use of vasoconstrictor medications and tobacco). It is good practice to estimate the tobacco consumption in pack years (for example, 20 cigarettes a day for one year equals one pack year).

PHYSICAL EXAMINATION AND TESTS

The physical examination should take particular note of the skin of the fingers, palms, wrists, and forearms to note any skin thickening (callus), laceration scars, and trophic changes. Abnormal muscular development or wasting should be noted together with any skeletal abnormalities.

To determine whether there is any thoracic outlet obstruction due to abnormal muscular development or deformity (for example, cervical rib), the *Adson's Test or maneuver*[6] should be conducted. With the patient sitting in a comfortable position, arms relaxed on thighs, the neck extended fully and the chin turned toward the side being examined, the patient is instructed to take a deep breath and hold it. A positive test includes production of symptoms or a pale hand; the radial pulse is diminished or lost. It is valuable to repeat the test with the head turned to the opposite side. In addition to Adson's test, the hyperabduction and costoclavicular maneuvers are worth doing. In the *hyperabduction maneuver,* while the radial pulse is continuously palpated with the patient sitting, the arm is slowly hyperabducted, (that is, it is raised above head level and rotated slightly away from the body). Production of symptoms or pallor of the hand constitute a positive test; the radial pulse is obliterated or diminished.

In the *costoclavicular maneuver* the patient, while sitting, pulls the shoulder backward and downward and holds a deep breath. Production of symptoms or pallor of the hand constitutes a positive test; the radial pulse is obliterated or diminished.

An additional test designed to detect the neurogenic component of the thoracic outlet syndrome (TOS) is the elevated-arms stress test, commonly referred to as the *abduction external rotation test.*[7-9] The subject sits erect and elevates both arms to the 90° abduction-external-rotation position with the elbows slightly braced back of the frontal plane ("holdup position"). The subject is asked to open and close his or her hands slowly for three minutes. The normal reaction is mild forearm tightness and deltoid and trapezius muscle fatigue. Patients with TOS develop progressive distress and reproduction of their usual symptoms (pain in the neck, shoulder, and/or arm; numbness and/or tingling of the extremity; heaviness, fatigue, and weakness of the arm and/or hand). A positive association is also reported in subjects exposed to vibrating tools and manual work.[10]

If any one of these maneuvers is positive, an x-ray of the cervical spine and upper rib cage is advisable.

Grip strength is evaluated with the use of a dynamometer. It is customary to record the best of two or more flexor contractions with each hand. Grip strength between subjects can vary considerably and normative age-related data for adults is available.[11] The results are more valuable and meaningful if they are repeated in a series of follow-up examinations.[12]

To detect circulatory lesions at or distal to the wrist, *Allen's test* should be performed.[13] While the examiner compresses both radial and ulnar arteries, the patient is asked to raise the hand and open and close the fist to drive the blood out of the vessels in the hand. The hand is then lowered and pressure on the radial artery is released. Prompt flushing of the hand is an indication that the artery, which has been released, contributes normally to the hand circulation. Faint and delayed flushing of more than five seconds to the digits indicates that the volar arches, or the digital arteries or the artery itself, at the wrist, are occluded. The process is repeated and the reaction checked on release of the ulnar artery.

The *Lewis-Prusik nail press test* may be used to detect impaired circulation to the peripheral vessels. Pressure is applied to the nail bed for ten seconds to occlude the circulation and produce a white nail bed. With normal circulation, recovery time is less than five seconds. All fingers may be tested, but normally one uses the middle finger unless another finger suffers more severely from Raynaud's phenomenon. At a room temperature of 20°C, this test has not been very useful in distinguishing Raynaud's phenomenon subjects from controls, but if performed after a one minute immersion in cold water at 4°C in a room temperature of 6°C, a statistically significant delay in recovery has been noted.[14]

For the detection of the carpal tunnel syndrome (CTS), which is often associated with HAVS, the Tinel and Phalen tests may be used. For the *Tinel test*, the subject's hand and forearm should be placed horizontally on a flat hard surface. A tendon hammer is used to tap the median nerve at the wrist, and the test is positive if symptoms of tingling are noticed in the innervated fingers.[15] In *Phalen's test* the patient's hands are raised to chin level and held in maximum wrist flexion for one minute. The test is positive if the right angle flexion of the wrist produces tingling of the innervated fingers. These tests unfortunately have low sensitivity and specificity.[16] Nerve-conduction velocity (NCV) tests are essential for confirmation of diagnosis.[17]

To evaluate skin sensitivity, an improved design of Renfrew's original esthesiometer[18] has been described by Carlson.[19] The *depth sense esthesiometer* has a surface containing a step of varying height, which slopes at a rate of 0.1 mm/cm horizontal distance. The total horizontal sensory length is 15 cm (normal tactile perception range 0 to 1.5 mm). The *two-point discrimination esthesiometer* has a surface containing a deep double-edged groove spreading at a rate of 0.4 mm/cm for 15 cm longitudinal length (normal tactile discrimination range 0 to 6.0 mm). Graduations in centimeters are engraved on the side of each esthesiometer. A constant finger pressure, position, and travel rate is required on the esthesiometer during the test. The upper normal limit for two-point discrimination is 3.2 mm [20-23] and the upper normal limit for depth sense appreciation is 0.50 mm.[24-28] The specificity of esthesiometric threshold testing is high. The sensitivity is better for depth sense than two-point discrimination.[29, 30] A vibration-free exposure interval of 18 hours before esthesiometric testing is important to avoid temporary threshold shifts.[31, 32]

Alternative esthesiometers include an altered Renfrew using a circular plastic disk[33] and a modified Carlson with speed, direction of movement, and finger pressure constantly controlled.[34]

The skin temperature of subjects may be recorded by the use of thermistor probes. *Finger skin temperatures in cold air* have been used for screening population groups because of the simplicity. While the digits are exposed to cold air, the time course of the skin temperature and the pattern of the change are noted.[35, 36] Cutaneous thermal discrimination may be tested using *Minnesota thermal disks*— made of copper, stainless steel, glass, and polyvinyl chloride,[37] or a thermo-esthesiometer.[38]

Nail fold capillary microscopy has been used for diagnosing Raynaud's phenomenon due to secondary causes. After the skin of the nail fold is cleansed with alcohol, a film of immersion oil is applied. The superficial blood vessels can then be visualized with a magnifying glass, ophthalmoscope, or a compound microscope with a cool light source. Normally, the superficial capillaries are seen as regularly spaced, hair pin loops aligned along the axis of the digit; the subpapillary venus plexus can be seen in fewer than 10 percent of subjects. Abnormalities consisting of enlarged and tortuous capillary loops, a sparsity of capillaries, and avascular areas may be seen in patients with connective tissue disease, particularly scleroderma, mixed connective tissue disease, and dermatomyositis.[39]

SPECIAL INVESTIGATIONS

Vascular

The use of *Doppler* ultrasonic instrumentation to record blood flow and to record the systolic pressures in the brachial, radial, and ulnar arteries is a very easy and useful laboratory test. *Digital blood pressure* measurement by photocell or strain gange plethysmography should be carried out at the intermediate phalanx of the fingers and the proximal phalanx of the thumb for higher diagnostic value. All digits should be measured, and the ratio of the digit systolic with the arm systolic pressure will give a good indication as to whether there is any impairment of digit blood flow (see Figure 5-1).

Using *photocell or strain gauge plethysmography*, the finger and toe pulse wave forms can be compared pre- and post-cold stress following immersion in water at 10°C for three minutes. Variations in *wave form pattern* may be detected, and the absence of a dicrotic notch with a slow up-stroke always indicates occlusive organic disease. Patients who suffer from vasospasm usually show a normal wave form at warm temperatures, but when exposed to cold, the wave forms become abnormal and may be completely flattened if there is severe spasm[40, 41] (see figures 5-2, 5-3, and 5-4).

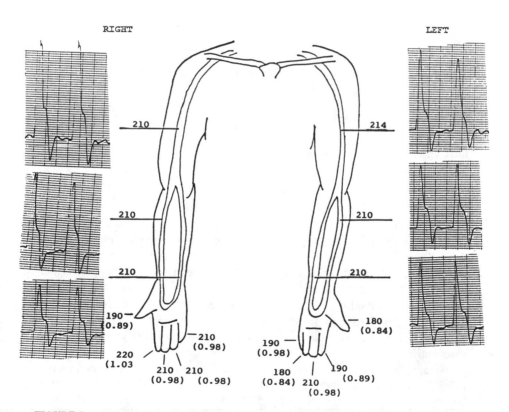

ARTERIAL PERIPHERAL STUDY – ARMS

FIGURE 5-1.   Doppler blood pressure measurements, arm-digit ratios and wave forms.

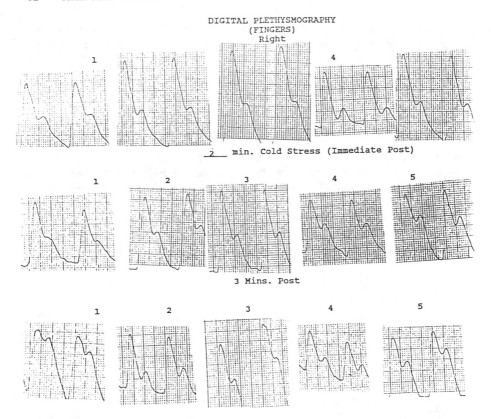

FIGURE 5-2.   Digital plethysmography fingers. Normal wave forms pre- and postcold stress.

Modifications of these procedures have been used by some researchers. These include photocell plethysmography while the opposite hand is immersed in ice water,[42] and measurement of blood flow responses in one hand while alternating thermal stimuli are applied to the contralateral hand.[43] Arterial blood flow measurements may be determined using a 20 MHz pulsed ultrasonic Doppler velocimeter,[44] while capillary blood flow in digits may be measured by the hydrogen gas clearance method using electrolysis[45] or xenon 133 washout technique.[46-72] Significant differences in flow rates distinguish subjects with and without Raynaud's phenomenon,[49] and flow rates can be used to identify vibration-elicited vasocontriction.[50]

Measurement of *digital blood pressure before and after local cooling* is a valuable vascular laboratory test.[51-55] The finger systolic blood pressure (FSBP) is measured with finger cooling to 30°C, 15°C and 10°C during five minutes ischemia. Using an FSBP percentage (10°C) of less than 60 percent as a discriminating

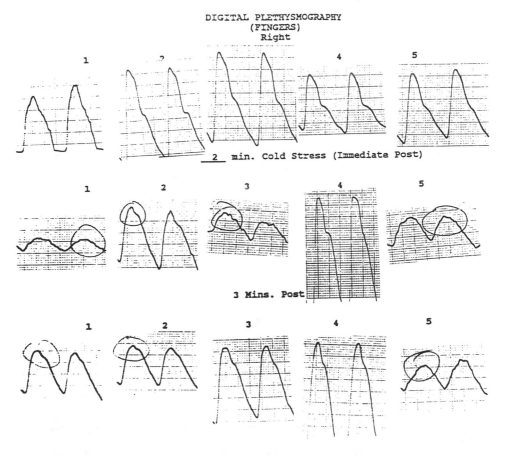

DIGITAL PLETHYSMOGRAPHY
(FINGERS)
Right

2 min. Cold Stress (Immediate Post)

3 Mins. Post

FIGURE 5-3.   Digital plethysmography fingers. Mild vasospasm postcold stress.

threshold between normals and patients with HAVS (stage 2 or more), the sensitivity of the cold test is 82 percent to 87 percent, and the specificity 90 percent to 100 percent.[56-58] If the response is not significant at room temperature, whole body cooling using a perfusion blanket at 10°C for 15 minutes should be used and the test repeated. If the blood pressure threshold is now significantly reduced, it indicates that the potential for vasospasm is less.[59]

A modification of the cold provocation test has been described using FSBP percentage at 15°C with body cooling for 15 minutes at a room temperature of 16°C. If normal, it is repeated at 10°C. The digital systolic blood pressure in the cooled test finger is calculated as a percentage of the systolic pressure in the arm (DP percentage) as opposed to the systolic pressure in a reference finger, (FSBP percentage). The two ways of calculating the test result give a similar sensitivity—

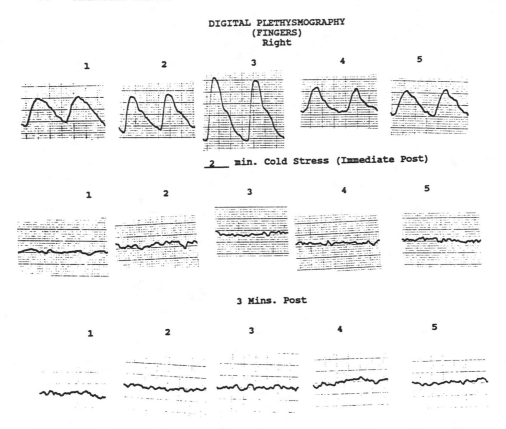

FIGURE 5-4.   Digital plethysmography fingers. Severe vasospasm postcold stress and dampened wave forms precold stress.

74 percent for FSBP percentage, and 79 percent for DP percentage.[60] Although the FSBP measurement test is not superior to cold provocation by whole-hand water immersion, it is being increasingly used since it is easier to standardize and more comfortable for the test subject.[61]

Cold-water immersion tests of the hands to record skin temperatures by thermisters before, during, and after immersion are useful both to confirm the presence of vasospasm and to grade its severity. Researchers have used water bath temperatures from 4°C to 15°C, and for immersion periods ranging from one to ten minutes.[62-69] Immersion at 10°C for ten minutes is the temperature and time for maximum patient tolerance and optimum results.

The thermisters have to be carefully calibrated for accuracy and must be applied to the tips of the digits with good skin contact. Threshold temperature recordings should be taken at room temperature for up to five minutes before immersing the hands (separately or both together). For the first five minutes, while immersed, the circulation at the wrists should be restricted with sphygmomanometer cuffs. The thermister readings need to be recorded at frequent intervals on a digital chart recorder or computer (see figures 5-5 to 5-8) and careful note should be taken of the digit temperatures at five minutes and ten minutes while immersed. The extent of any reactive hyperemia, occurring while immersed when the sphygmomanometer cuffs are released at five minutes, should be noted. Following immersion, the hands should be carefully dried to reduce evaporative cooling and the thermister recordings followed for at least ten minutes. The test is normally conducted at room temperature or with the patient wrapped in a blanket at 35°C. By noting the digit temperatures reached during immersion, the extent of the reactive hyperemia if any, and the recovery time following immersion, vasospasm may be diagnosed and its severity graded.[70-75] The sensitivity and specificity of this test is over 90 percent.[76, 77]

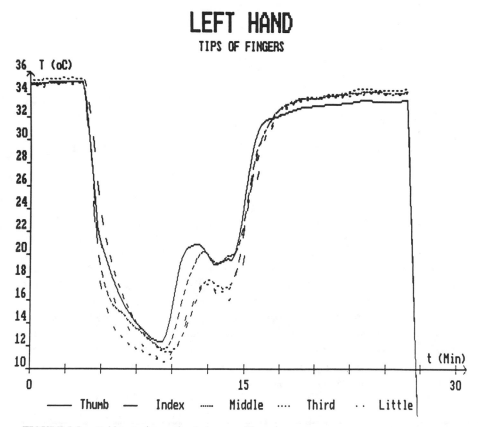

FIGURE 5-5.   Cold-water immersion test curves. Normal response.

RIGHT HAND
TIPS OF FINGERS

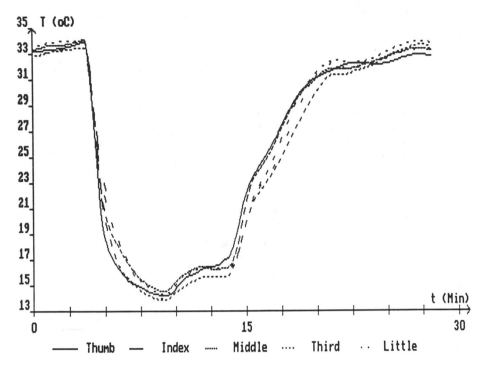

FIGURE 5-6.   Cold-water immersion test curves. Mild vasospasm.

By evaluating the results of the Doppler, plethysmography, FSBP, and cold-water immersion tests, vasospasm of the digits may be reliably diagnosed and graded in severity. Stage I (mild) requires a positive cold-water immersion and/or Doppler test. Stage 2 (moderate) requires a more severe positive cold-water immersion test and in addition a positive FSBP percentage test with blanket cooling. Stage 3 (severe) requires, together with a severe positive cold-water immersion test, a positive FSBP percentage test without the cooling blanket.

Infrared thermography may be used to assess skin temperature during cold provocation tests, but considering the expense, it has little to offer and it does not match the accuracy of fingertip thermometry. It is only relevant for special clinical work,[73, 79] since the results are often equivocal.[80]

Brachial arteriography has been used to evaluate HAV subjects. It is preferable to use noninvasive methods. Its use should be restricted for the diagnosis of organic vascular lesions.[81-83]

RIGHT HAND
TIPS OF FINGERS

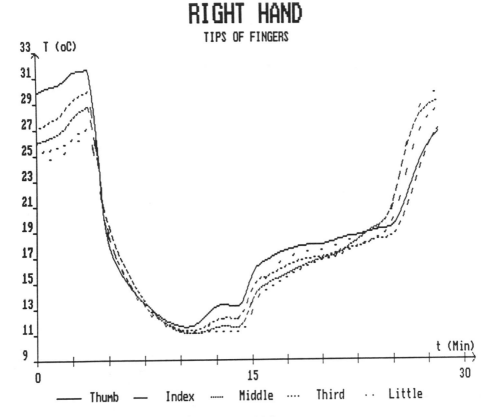

FIGURE 5-7.   Cold-water immersion test curves. Moderate vasospasm.

Neurological

Vibration perception thresholds to single frequencies (for example, 100 Hz), may be determined at the fingertips using hand-held vibrometers (biothesiometers)[84, 85] and they have been used in field studies.[86, 87] If there is no direct control of applied pressure there will be operator and technique variability. Vibrometers are now available to evaluate vibration perception over the frequency range 8 to 500 Hz, at constant pressure,[88-91] and are being increasingly used to monitor subjects with known CTS complicated by HAVS.[92, 93]

The factors influencing vibration sensory thresholds include: contact force, contactor probe diameter, the surround contour and its diameter around the probe, test frequencies, and temporary threshold shifts.[94] Although it is a test dependent on subjective response, if the subject is cooperative, the vibrogram can be a reliable clinical assessment when an initial practice trial is included as part of the standard program.[95]

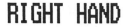

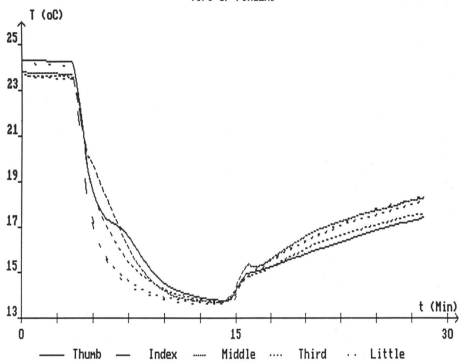

FIGURE 5-8.   Cold-water immersion test curves. Severe vasospasm.

Investigations in the early 1920s showed that HAVS subjects had reduced appreciation of skin temperature. This was identified by their ability to handle hot objects and materials, which sometimes resulted in burns to the digits. This observation lead to the development of *thermal detection threshold tests.* Such a test will define temperature appreciation—cold and hot zones—and determine at the same time thermal pain thresholds for each digit. The subject rests the pulp of a digit on a metal plate (35mm × 40mm), the temperature of which is controlled. The rate of temperature change is 10°C per second and the subject presses a switch whenever a warm/cold sensation is experienced.[96]

Current perception threshold testing is being increasingly used to evaluate sensorineural impairment. Current perception thresholds (CPTs) are obtained using a neurometer. This portable, battery operated (6V) device generates a graded sinusoid at 5, 250, and 2,000 Hz with a constant current from 0 to 10 milliamperes. The current is delivered to the skin surface in short stimuli (2–5s) via a pair of 1 cm in diameter gold electrodes separated by 1.7 cm and covered by a thin layer of electrode paste. The detection thresholds at each frequency are determined for the median and ulnar nerves on two digits. An advantage is that the test may be conducted over a wide range of skin temperatures and on edemetous skin. This subjective test evaluates the integrity of sensory afferents, and the results correlate significantly with nerve conduction test findings.[97-100] Because the intensity thresholds for perception are very different at the different test frequencies it has been suggested that CPT is able to evaluate selectively three specific populations of the axons in a peripheral nerve. The high-frequency detection thresholds correlate best with tests of large fiber function and the low frequency with small fiber function. The most frequently applied test of small fiber (C fiber) function has been to determine thermal detection and pain thresholds from 10 to 15°C using, for example, a thermotest apparatus with a solid-state heat pump. It has been demonstrated by microneurography that C fibers in human skin can be stimulated electronically at low frequencies, so a CPT test at 5 Hz is preferable. That CPT gives information about the functional integrity of different fiber types is suggested by the correlation with thermal (5 Hz) and vibration (250 Hz) testing.

It is by no means certain that transcutaneous current stimulates nerve endings directly. It may be that the differential responses of cutaneous mechanoreceptors to different frequencies of mechanical stimulation is the mechanism by which different sensations are evoked. All tests for evaluating sensory function are not measuring nerve function specifically. Interpretation of results in this way always assumes the integrity of central sensory pathways.[101]

Nerve-conduction velocity testing is the most widely used quantitative neurophysiological tool for evaluating peripheral neuropathy. The objective testing of the peripheral nerve is very advantageous as it eliminates the reporting bias in subjective tests. But it is important to appreciate that convential electrodiagnostic studies primarily assess the function of somatic motor axons and large-diameter sensory fibers. Their diagnostic utility is thus limited in conditions that selectively affect autonomic or small-diameter fibers. The standard motor or sensory conduction velocity measures the conducting capacity of the largest, myelinated, rapidly conducting fibers in the nerve. Hence, the velocity is most clearly abnormal when the myelin sheath is disrupted. Amplitude and duration of the evoked potential are equally important in establishing a diagnosis. A decrease in amplitude reflects either loss of axons or loss of muscle fibers, or may indicate a conduction block.[102, 103] Nerve-conduction velocity is affected by age and temperature, and scrupulously careful techniques must be used by technicians to ensure accurate, meaningful results.

This test is essential to confirm sensorineural impairment from HAV exposure[104] and the presence of CTS,[105, 106] a condition often associated with HAVS. It can also identify compression neuropathy of the ulnar nerve.[107]

Needle electromyography (EMG) is an invasive test since a thin needle has to be inserted into the muscle belly. The EMG records the physical activity within the muscle, yielding information about its resting state, about activity when the muscle contracts, and indirectly about the condition of the nerve enervating the muscle. When nerve fibers are demyelinated but the axons remain, the number of motor units recruited during voluntary contraction is reduced. There is no abnormal activity in the resting state. When axonal degeneration occurs, denervation also occurs, yielding alterations in the behaviour of muscle fibers at rest and during contraction. It is rarely necessary to use this test for HAV-exposed patients.

Somatosensory evoked potentials (SEPs) are elicited by applying a brief electric current to the skin overlying a peripheral nerve. Cortical SEPs are of maximal amplitude in the central region of the brain, contralateral to the site of stimulation. Their component make up and scalp topography has been extensively character-ized.[108] Because of the time and the expensive equipment required to administer SEPs, the expertise required to interpret them, and their status as relative newcom-ers in neurotoxicity testing, evoked potentials must presently be considered as research tools awaiting further development.

To evaluate manipulative dexterity, several tests are available. The *Purdue pegboard* measures dexterity for two types of activity: one involving gross movements of hands, fingers, and arms; and the other involving primarily what might be called fingertip dexterity. The pegboard is equipped with pins, collars, and washers and is a test to see how quickly and accurately they can be assembled.

The *Moberg pick-up test* requires the subject to pick up a series of 10 to 12 small objects of various sizes from a table surface and place them in a small container. It may be adapted to include recognition variables.[109] A modified pick-up test has been described by Dellon, which requires increasing discrimination for object recognition.[110]

Objective *sweat tests* based on the fact that there is a direct relationship between the sensory supply to the skin and the sympathetic supply to the sweat glands in the same area of skin include:

a. the *wrinkle test*.[111] In this test the hands are immersed in water at 40°c for a period of 30 minutes, and the normal shrivelling of the skin of the fingers is observed. Denervated skin does not shrivel; it remains smooth.

b. the *Moberg ninhydrin test*[112] relies on the characteristic color reaction of ninhydrin with the amino acids present in sweat. The pulps of the digits are applied to dry, nonporous paper, which is then immersed in 1 percent ninhydrin solution in acetone. On heating (100°C to 120°C for 5 to 10 minutes in an oven), the fingerprints become visible, and the result is read in terms of colored dots. It is conclusive only when the dots are absent in the denervated area.

c. an alternate to ninhydrin is 2 percent to 3 percent *bromphenol blue* solution.[113] Paper soaked in it becomes orange-yellow. When dry the pulps of the digits are applied, and the sweat dots appear as deep blue. Although the dots are more legible than with ninhydrin and the test is objective, it is unfortunately qualitative not quantitative. When there is sensorineural impairment, as in HAVS patients, sweat tests are not helpful in quantifying the severity.

For sensorineural severity stage 1 SN (mild) some subjective tests may or may not be positive. For stage 2 SN (moderate) there has to be reduced sensory perception, and most tests should be positive including thermal detection and/or current perception threshold. For stage 3 SN (severe) there is usually persistent numbness, reduced tactile discrimination and/or reduced manipulation dexterity. The nerve condition test should also be positive.

Audiometry to determine hearing thresholds over the frequency range 250 Hz through 8,000 Hz should be conducted using manual or self-recording audiometry. The subject should have a noise-free interval of at least 18 hours prior to the test. Noise-induced hearing loss will be evident if there is an elevated threshold at 4,000 Hz and the loss is diagnosed as sensorineural. Evoked-response audiometry should be reserved for compensation cases when there is doubt regarding the subjective test result.

SUMMARY

The clinical evaluation of a patient with HAVS will vary according to the purpose of the examination. The medical and occupational history is always required, but selection of tests will be dependent on the personal preference of the physician and the laboratory facilities available. Both screening and special investigation tests appropriate for the vascular and sensorineural assessment of such patients are reviewed. Doppler, digital systolic blood pressure, and cold-water immersion tests are the vascular laboratory tests most favored, while nerve-conduction, thermal detection, and current perception threshold tests are preferred for sensorineural evaluation. A combination of the test results will determine the severity by stage of the vascular and sensorineural components of each hand. A summary of appropriate tests is given in Appendix 1.

Notes
1. Pelmear P. L. "Clinical Evaluation of Vibration-Exposed Complainants in Field Surveys." *Scand. J. Work Environ. Health* 1987; 13:284–285.
2. Ekenvall, L. "Clinical Assessment of Suspected Damage From Hand-Held Vibrating Tools." *Scand. J. Work. Environ. Health* 1987; 13:271–274.
3. Pyykkö, I. "Clinical Aspects of the Hand-Arm Vibration Syndrome. A Review." *Scand. J. Work. Environ. Health* 1986; 12:439–447.

92   Hand-Arm Vibration

4. Matoba, T. and Sakurai, T. "Diagnosis of Peripheral Circulatory Functions in Vibration Disease." *Japanese J. Trauma Occup. Med.* 1985; 33(5):357-367.
5. Pelmear, P. L., and Taylor, W. "Hand-Arm Vibration Syndrome—Clinical Evaluation and Prevention." *J. Occup. Med.* (in Press).
6. Adson, A. W. "Surgical Treatment for Symptoms Produced by Cervical Ribs and the Scalenus Anticus Muscle." *Surg. Gynecol. Obstet.* 1947; 85:687-700.
7. Ross, D. "Congenital Anomalies Associated With Thoracic Outlet Syndrome." *Amer. J. Surg.* 1976; 132:771-778.
8. Roos, D. "Pathophysiology of Congenital Anomalies in Thoracic Outlet Syndrome." *Acta. Chir. Belg.* 1980; 5:353-361.
9. Pang, D. and Wessel, H. B. "Thoracic Outlet Syndrome." *Neurosurgery* 1988; 22(1):105-121.
10. Toomingas, A.; Hagberg, M.; Jorulf, L.; Nilsson, T.; Burström, L.; Kihlberg, S. "Outcome of the Abduction External Rotation Test Among Manual and Office Workers." *Amer. J. Ind. Med.* 1991; 19:215-227.
11. Mathiowetz, Ms, Kashman, N.; Volland, G.; Weber, K.; Dowe, M.; Rogers, S. "Grip and Pinch Strength: Normative Data for Adults." *Arch. Phys. Med. Rehabil.* 1985; 66:69-74.
12. Färkkilä, M.; Aatola, S.; Stark, J.; Korhonen, O.; Pyykkö, I. "Hand-Grip Force in Lumberjacks: Two-Year Follow-up." *Int. Arch. Occup. Environ. Health* 1986; 58:203-208.
13. Ashbell, T. S.; Kutz, J. E.; Kleinert, H. E. "The Digital Allen Test." *Plast. Reconstr. Surg.* 1967; 39:311-312.
14. Okada, A.; Yamashita, T.; Ideda, T. "Screening Test for Raynaud's Phenomenon of Occupational Origin." *Amer. Ind. Hyg. Assoc. J.* 1972; 476-482.
15. Mossman, S. S., and Blau, J. N. "Tinels Sign and the Carpal Tunnel Syndrome." *BMJ* 1987; 294:680.
16. Heller, L.; Ring, H.; Costeff, H.; Solzi, P. "Evaluation of Tinel's and Phalen's Signs in Diagnosis of the Carpal Tunnel Syndrome." *Ear Neurol.* 1986; 25:40-42.
17. De Krom, M. C. T. F. M.; Knipschild, P. G.; Kester, A. D. M.; Spaars, F. "Efficacy of Provocative Tests for Diagnosis of Carpal Tunnel Syndrome." *Lancet* 1990; 335:393-395.
18. Renfrew, S. "Fingertip Sensation: A Routine Neurological Test." *Lancet* 1969; 1:396-397.
19. Carlson, W. S.; Samueloff, S.; Taylor, W.; Wassermann, D. E. "Instrumentation for Measurement of Sensory Loss in the Fingertips." *J. Occup. Med.* 1979; 21(4):260-264.
20. Bovenzi, M., and Zadini, A. "Quantitative Estimation of Aesthesiometric Thresholds for Assessing Impaired Tactile Sensation in Workers Exposed to Vibration." *Int. Arch. Occup. Environ. Health* 1989; 61:431-435.
21. Carlson, W.; Smith, R.; Taylor, W. "Vibration Syndrome in Chipping and Grinding Workers: V.A. Aesthesiometry." *J. Occup. Med.* 1984; 26:776-780.
22. Pelmear, P. L.; Taylor, W.; Pearson, J. C. G. "Clinical Objective Tests for Vibration White Finger." In: Taylor, W. and Pelmear, P. L. eds. *Vibration White Finger in Industry.* New York: Academic Press, 1975; 396-397.
23. Brammer, A. J.; Taylor, W.; Piercy, J. E. "Assessing the Severity of Neurological Component of the Hand-Arm Vibration Syndrome." *Scand. J. Work. Environ. Health* 1986; 12:427-431.

24. Bovenzi and Zadini, "Quantitative Estimation."
25. Carlson, Smith, and Taylor, "Vibration Syndrome."
26. Pelmear, Taylor, and Pearson, "Clinical Objective Tests."
27. Brammer, Taylor, and Piercy, "Assessing the Severity."
28. Haines, T. and Chong, J. P. "Peripheral Neurological Assessment Methods for Workers Exposed to Hand-Arm Vibration. An Appraisal." *Scand. J. Work. Environ. Health* 1987; 13:370–374.
29. Ibid.
30. Pelmear, Taylor, and Pearson, "Clinical Objective Tests."
31. Haines, T.; Chong, J.; Verrall, A. B.; Julian, J.; Bernholz, C.; Spears, R.; Muir, D. C. F. "Aesthisiometric Threshold Changes Over the Course of Workshift in Miners Exposed to Hand-Arm Vibration." *Brit. J. Ind. Med.* 1988; 45:106–111.
32. Verbeck, M. M.; Salle, H. J. A.; Kempers, O. "Vibratory and Tactile Sense of the Fingers After Working With Sanders." *Int. Arch. Occup. Environ. Health* 1985; 56:217–223.
33. Sivayoganathan, K.; Akinmayowa, N. K.; Corlett, E. N. "Objective Test for the Vibration Syndrome and Reduction of Vibration During Fettling." In: Brammer, A. T. and Taylor, W., eds. Vibration Effects on the Hand and Arm in Industry. New York: John Wiley & Sons, 1982; 325–331.
34. Chatterjee, D. S. "A New Depth-Sense Esthesiometer." *Scand. J. Work. Environ. Health* 1987; 13:323–325.
35. Fritz, M. "Computer-Aided Evaluation of Schwarzlose's Cold Air Test for the Diagnosis of Vibration Induced White Finger Disease. *Zbl Arbeitsmed* 1984; 39: 94–99 (English Summary).
36. Tanaka, I.; Inoue, N.; Akiyama, T. "Peripheral Circulation Analyzer for Diagnosis of Vibration Syndrome." In: Okada, A.; Taylor, W.; Dupuis, H. *Hand-Arm Vibration.* Kanazawa, Japan: Kyoei Press, 1990; 191–193.
37. Dyck, P. J.; Curtis, D. J.; Bushek, W.; Offord, K. "Description of Minnesota Thermal Dices and Normal Values of Thermal Discrimination in Man." *Neurology* 1974; 24(4):325–330.
38. Hirosawa, I. "Original Construction of Thermo-Esthesiometer and Its Application to Vibration Disease." *Int. Arch. Environ. Health* 1983; 52:209–214.
39. Maricq, H. R.; LeRoy, E. C.; D'Angelo, W. A.; Medsger, T. A.; Rodnan, G. P.; Sharp, G. G.; Wolfe, J. F. "Diagnostic Potential of in vivo Capillary Microscopy in Scleroderma and Related Disorders." *Arthritis Rheum.* 1980; 23(2):183–189.
40. Holmgren, R. N.; Baur, G. M.; Porter, J. M. "Vascular Laboratory Evaluation of Raynaud's Syndrome." *Bruit* 1981; V:19–22.
41. Hirai, M. "Arterial Insufficiency of the Hand Evaluated by Digital Blood Pressure and Arteriographic Findings." *Circulation* 1978; 58(5): 902–908.
42. Samuelhoff, S.; Miday, R.; Wasserman, D.; Behrens, V.; Hornung, R.; Asburry, W.; Doyle, T.; Dukes-Dobos, F.; Badger, D. "A Peripheral Vascular Insufficiency Test Using Photocell Plethysmography." *J. Occup. Med.* 1981; 23(9):643–646.
43. Lafferty, K.; De Trafford, J. C.; Roberts, V. C.; Cotton, L. T. "Raynaud's Phenomenon and Thermal Entrainment: An Objective Test." *BMJ* 1983; 286:90–92.
44. Brown, T. D., Blair; W. F., Gabel; R. H., Morecraft; R. J. "Effects of Episodic Air Hammer Usage on Digital Artery Haemodynamics of Foundry Workers With Vibration White Finger Disease." *J. Occup. Med.* 1988; 30(ii):853–862.

45. Aukland, A.; Bower, B. F.; Berliner, R. W. "Measurement of Local Blood Flow With Hydrogen Gas." *Circ. Res.* 1964; 14:164–187.
46. Sejrsen, P. "Blood Flow in Cutaneous Tissue in Man Studied by Washout of Radioactive Xenon." *Circulat. Res.* 1969; 25:215–229.
47. Sejrsen, P. "Atraumatic Local Labelling of Skin by Inert Gas: Epicutaneous Application of Xenon 133." *J. Appl. Physiol.* 1968; 24:570–572.
48. Olsen, N. and Petring, O. U. "Vibration Elicited Vasoconstrictor Reflex in Raynaud's Phenomena." *Brit. J. Ind. Med.* 1988; 45:415–419.
49. Okada, A. and Nohara, S. "Studies on the Finger Blood Flow and Peripheral Nerve Conduction Velocity in Workers Using Vibrating Tools." In: See, L. C.; Fook, L. W.; Peng, L. H.; Nam, O. C., eds. "Proceedings of the 10th Asian Conference on Occupational Health." Singapore 1982; 1:408–410.
50. Olsen, N.; Petring, O. U.; Rossing, N. "Transitory Postural Vasomotor Dysfunction in the Finger After Short Term Hand Vibration." *Brit. J. Ind. Med.* 1989; 46:575–581.
51. Olsen, N.; Nielson, S. L.; Voss, P. "Cold Response of Digital Arteries in Chain Saw Operators." *Brit. J. Ind. Med.* 1981; 38:82–88.
52. Ekenvall, L. and Lindblad, L. E. "Digital Blood Pressure After Local Working as a Diagnostic Tool in Traumatic Vasopastic Disease." *Brit. J. Ind. Med.* 1982; 39:388–391.
53. Gates, K. H.; Tyburczy, J. A.; Zupan, T.; Baur, G. M.; Porter, J. M. "The Non-Invasive Quantification of Digital Vasospasm." *BRUIT* 1984; 34–37.
54. Arneklo-Nobin, B.; Johansen, K.; Sjoberg, T. "The Objective Diagnosis of Vibration-Induced Vascular Injury." *Scand. J. Work. Environ. Health* 1987; 13:337–342.
55. Bovenzi, M. "Vibration White Finger, Digital Blood Pressure, and Some Biochemical Findings on Workers Operating Vibrating Tools in the Engine Manufacturing Industry." *Amer. J. Occup. Med.* 1988; 14:575–584.
56. Bovenzi, M. "Finger Systolic Pressure During Local Cooling in Normal Subjects Aged 20–60 Years: Reference Values for the Assessment of Digital Vasospasm in Raynaud's Phenomenon of Occupational Origin." *Int. Arch. Occup. Environ. Health* 1988; 61:179–181.
57. Bovenzi, M. "Vibration Exposure, Vibration-Induced White Finger and Digital Arterial Tone in Chain Saw Operators." *J. Low Freq. Noise Vib.* 1991; 10(1):15–25.
58. Kurozawa, Y.; Nasu, Y.; Nose, T. "Diagnostic Value of Finger Systolic Blood Pressure in the Assessment of Vasospastic Reactions in the Finger Skin of Vibration-Exposed Subjects After Finger and Body Cooling." *Scand. J. Work. Environ. Health.* 1991; 17:184–189.
59. Ibid.
60. Ekenvall, L.; Lindblad, L. E. "Vibration White Finger and Digital Systolic Pressure During Cooling." *Brit. J. Ind. Med.* 1986; 43:280–283.
61. Pyykkö, I.; Färkkilä, M.; Korhonen, O.; Stark, J.; Jäntti, V. "Cold Provocation Tests in the Evaluation of Vibration-Induced White Finger." *Scand. J. Work. Environ. Health* 1986; 12:254–258.
62. Kurozawa, Nasu, and Nose, "Diagnostic Value."
63. Pyykkö, Färkkilä, Korhonen; Stark; and Jäntti, "Cold Provocation Tests."
64. Juul, C. and Nielson, S. L. "Locally Induced Digital Vasospasm Detected by Delayed Rewarming in Raynaud's Phenomenon of Occupational Origin." *Brit. J. Ind. Med.* 1981; 38:87–90.

65. Pelmear, P. L.; Roos, J.; Leong, D.; Wong, L. "Cold Provocation Test Results From a 1985 Survey of Hard Rock Miners in Ontario." *Scand. J. Work. Environ. Health* 1987; 13:343–347.

66. Pelmear, P. L.; Taraschuk, I.; Leong, D.; Wong, L. "Cold Water Immersion Test in Hand-Arm Vibration Exposed." *J. Low Freq. Noise Vib.* 1985; 4(3):89–97.

67. Miyashita, K.; Takeda, S.; Kasamatsu, T.; Hashimoto, T.; Iwata, H. "Cold Water Immersion Test (1 Minute Immersion in 4°C Water) and Its Evaluation." In: Okada, A.; Taylor, W.; Dupuis, H., eds. *Hand-Arm Vibration.* Kanazawa, Japan: Kyoei Press, 1990:211–214.

68. Ishitake, T.; Ohkubo, A.; Oki, M.; Suenaga, T.; Sakurai, T.; Matoba, T. "A Simplified Cold Water Immersion Test for Peripheral Circulatory Function." In: Okada, A.; Taylor, W.; Dupuis, H., eds. *Hand-Arm Vibration.* Kanazawa, Japan: Kyoei Press, 1990:215–219.

69. Welsh, C. L. "Digital Rewarming Time in the Assessment of Vibration-Induced White Finger." *Scand. J. Work. Environ. Health* 1986; 12:249–250.

70. Pelmear, Roos, Leong, and Wong, "Cold Provocation Test."

71. Pelmear, Taraschuk, Leong, and Wong, "Cold Water Immersion."

72. Miyashita, Takeda, Kasamatsu, Hashimoto, and Iwata. "Cold Water Immersion Test."

73. Ishitake, Ohkubo, Oki, Suenaga, Sakurai, Matoba, "Simplified Cold Water."

74. Welsh, "Digital Rewarming."

75. Hack, M.; Boillat, M. A.; Schweizer, C.; Lob, M. "Assessment of Vibration Induced White Finger: Reliability and Validity of Two Tests." *Brit. J. Ind. Med.* 1986; 43:284–287.

76. Niioka, T.; Kojima, Y.; Kaji, H.; Saito, K. "Diagnostic Method for Vibration Syndrome With Special Reference to Finger Skin Temperature and Vibratory Sense Threshold." *Scand. J. Work. Environ. Health* 1986; 12:251–253.

77. Kurumatani, N.; Iki, M.; Hirata, K.; Moriyama, T.; Satoh, M.; Arai, T. "Usefulness of Fingertip Stem Temperature for Examining Peripheral Circulatory Disturbances of Vibrating Tool Operators." *Scand. J. Work. Environ. Health* 1986; 12:245–248.

78. Bovenzi, M. "Finger Thermometry in the Assessment of Subjects With Vibration-Induced White Finger." *Scand. J. Work. Environ. Health* 1987; 13:348–351.

79. Dupuis, H. "Thermographic Assessment of Skin Temperature During a Cold Provocation Test." *Scand. J. Work. Environ. Health* 1987; 13:352–355.

80. Williams, D. M. J.; Robert, E.; Evans, K. T. "An Assessment of Hand Thermography in Vinyl Chloride Workers." *J. Soc. Occup. Med.* 1977; 27:57–62.

81. James, P. B. and Galloway, R. W. "Arteriography of the Hand in Men Exposed to Vibration." In: Taylor, W and Pelmear, P. L., eds. *Vibration White Finger in Industry.* London: Academic Press, 1975:31–41.

82. Arneklo-Nobin, B.; Edvinsson, L.; Eklof, B.; Haffajee, D.; Owman, C. H.; Thylen, U. "Analysis of Vasospasm in Hand Arteries by in vitro Pharmacology, Hand Angiography and Finger Plethysmography." *Gen. Pharmac.* 1983; 14:65–67.

83. Falappa, P.; Magnavita, N.; Bergamaschi, A.; Colavita, N. "Angiographic Study of Digital Arteries in Workers Exposed to Vinyl Chloride." *Brit. J. Ind. Med.* 1982; 39:169–172.

84. Wiles, P. G.; Pearce, S. M.; Rice, P. J. S.; Mitchell, J. M. O. "Reduced Vibration Perception in Right Hands of Normal Subjects: An Acquired Abnormality?" *Brit. J. Ind. Med.* 1990; 47:715–716.

85. Ekenvall, L.; Nilsson, B. Y.; Falconer, C. "Sensory Perception in the Hands of Dentists." *Scand. J. Environ. Health* 1990; 16:334-339.
86. Cherniack, M. G.; Letz, R; Gerr, F; Brammer, A; Pace, P. "Detailed Clinical Assessment of Neurological Function in Symptomatic Shipyard Workers." *Brit. J. Ind. Med.* 1990; 47:566-572.
87. Bove, F. J.; Letz, R.; Baker, E. L. "Sensory Thresholds Among Construction Trade Painters: A Cross-Sectional Study Using New Methods for Measuring Temperature and Vibration Sensitivity." *J. Occup. Med.* 1989; 31(4):320-325.
88. Lumborg, G.; Sollerman, C.; Stromberg, T.; Pyykkö, I.; Rosen, B. "A New Principle for Assessing Vitrotactile Sense in Vibration-Induced Neuropathy." *Scand. J. Work. Environ. Health* 1987; 13:375-379.
89. Aatola, S.; Färkkilä, M.; Pyykkö, I.; Korhonen, O.; Starck, J. "Measuring Method for Vibration Perception Threshold of Fingers and Its Application to Vibration Exposed Workers." *Int. Arch. Occup. Environ. Health* 1990; 62:239-242.
90. Grunert, B. K.; Wertsch, J. J.; Matloub, H. S.; McCallum-Burke, S. "Reliability of Sensory Threshold Measurement Using a Digital Vibrogram." *J. Occup. Med.* 1990; 32(2):100-102.
91. Lundstrom, R. "Digital Tactilogram as a Diagnostic Tool for Early Diagnosis of Vibration Induced Neuropathy." In: Okada, A.; Taylor, W.; Dupuis, H., eds. *Hand-Arm Vibration*. Kanazawa, Japan: Kyoei Press, 1990:75-72.
92. Jetzer, T. C.; MacLeod, D.; Conrad, J.; Troyer, S.; Jacobs, P.; Albin, T. "The Use of Vibration Testing to Evaluate Workers and Tools." In: Okada, A.; Taylor, W.; Dupuis, H., eds. *Hand-Arm Vibration*. Kanazawa, Japan: Kyoei Press, 1990:79-82.
93. Jetzer, C. J. "Use of Vibration Testing in the Early Evaluation of Workers With Carpal Tunnel Syndrome." *J. Occup. Med.* 1991; 33(2):117-120.
94. Harada, N. and Griffin, M. J. "Factors Influencing Vibration Sense Thresholds Used to Assess Occupational Exposures to Hand Transmitted Vibration." *Brit. J. Ind. Med.* 1991; 48:185-192.
95. Lundstrom, "Digital Tactilogram."
96. Ekenvall, L.; Nilsson, B. Y.; Gustavsson, P. "Temperature and Vibration Thresholds in Vibration Syndrome." *Brit. J. Ind. Med.* 1986; 43:825-829.
97. Katims, J. J.; Naviasky, E. H.; Randell, M. S.; Ng, L. K. Y.; Bleecker, M. L. "Constant Current Sine Wave Transcutaneous Nerve Stimulation for the Evaluation of Peripheral Neuropathy." *Arch. Phy. Med. Rehab.* 1987; 68:210-213.
98. Katims, J. J.; Naviasky, E. H.; Rendell, M. S.; Ng, L. K. Y.; Bleecker, M. L. "New Screening Device for Assessment of Peripheral Neuropathy." *J. Occup. Med.* 1986; 28(12):1219-1221.
99. Weseley, S. A.; Sadler, B.; Katims, J. J. "Current Perception Preferred Test for Evaluation of Peripheral Nerve Integrity." *Trans. Am. Soc. Artif. Intern. Organs* 1988; XXXIV:188-193.
100. Katims, J. J.; Rouvelas, P.; Sadler, B. T.; Weseley, S. A. "Current Perception Threshold: Reproducibility and Comparison With Nerve Conduction in Evaluation of Carpal Tunnel Syndrome." *Trans. Am. Soc. Artif. Intern. Organs* 1989; XXXV: 280-284.
101. Masson, E. A.; Veves, A.; Fernando, D.; Boulton, A. J. M. "Current Perception Thresholds: A New, Quick and Reproducable Method for the Assessment of Peripheral Neuropathy in Diabetes Mellitus." *Diabetologia* 1989; 32:724-728.

102. Moody, L.; Arezzo, J.; Otto, D. "Screening Occupational Populations for Asymptomatic or Early Peripheral Neuropathy." *J. Occup. Med.* 1986; 28(10):975–986.

103. Joynt, R. L. "Correlation Studies of Velocity, Amplitude, and Duration in Median Nerves." *Arch. Phys. Med. Rehabil.* 1989; 70:477–481.

104. Araki, S.; Yokoyama, K.; Aono, H.; Murata, K. "Determination of the Distribution of Nerve Conduction Velocities in Chain Saw Operators." *Brit. J. Ind. Med.* 1988; 45:341–344.

105. Golding, D. N.; Rose, D. M.; Selvarajah, K. "Clinical Tests for Carpal Tunnel Syndrome: An Evaluation." *Brit. J. Rheum.* 1986; 25:388–390.

106. Jackson, D. A.; and Clifford, J.C. "Electrodiagnosis of Mild Carpal Tunnel Syndrome." *Arch. Phys. Med. Rehabil.* 1989; 70:199–204.

107. Streib, E. W.; Sun, S. F. "Distal Ulnar Neuropathy in Meat Packers: An Occupational Disease?" *J. Occup. Med.* 1984; 26(11):842–843.

108. Goff, G.D.; Matsumiya, Y; Allison, T. et al. "The Scalp Topography of Human Somatosensory and Auditory Evoked Potentials." *Electroencephalogr. Clin. Neurophysiol.* 1977; 42:57–76.

109. Moberg, E. "Objective Method for Determining the Functional Value of Sensitivity in the Hand." *J. Bone. Joint. Surg.* 1958; 40(B):454–476.

110. Dellon, A. L., ed. "Evaluation of Sensibility and Re-education of Sensation in the Hand." Baltimore: Williams and Wilkin, 1981:95–113.

111. O'Riain, S. "New and Simple Test of Nerve Function in Hand." *BMJ* 1973:615–616.

112. Moberg, "Objective Method."

113. Sakurai, M. "Use of Bromphenol Blue Printing Method for Detecting Sweat in the Palm." *J. Hand. Surgery* 1986; 11(B):125–130.

6

Treatment and Management

P. L. Pelmear, W. Taylor

TREATMENT

Until recently, little effective progress had been made in the treatment of patients with hand-arm vibration syndrome (HAVS). This is shown by the numerous treatments advanced in the literature.

Initially physiotherapy involving balneotherapy (swimming pool), thermotherapy (hot packs), paraffin baths, contrast temperature baths, infrared and low-frequency therapy were popular forms of therapy and still are to a large extent in Japan.[1, 2] These therapies are palliative, but do result in subjective and psychological improvement.

Recent advances in treatment have focused on three aspects: (1) use of calcium channel antagonists to produce peripheral vasodilatation, (2) drugs to reduce platelet aggregation and adhesiveness, and (3) drugs to reduce blood viscosity and emboli formation.

Vasodilators

These drugs cause dilatation of blood vessels either by direct action on the musculature or by blocking the activity of alpha-adrenoreceptors in the vessel wall. They should be prescribed for subjects at stage 2 (Stockholm) who cannot avoid further exposure, and for ex-vibration-exposed workers with symptoms. Unfortunately, if given in sufficient dosage, or if the dosage is increased too quickly, the agent may raise the cardiac output or lower the blood pressure to such an extent that headache, ataxia, and syncope may occur. Mild to moderate peripheral edema has been reported. Symptoms of nausea and vomiting, gastrointestinal distress, flushing, and heat sensation have been documented. Some subjects may have

98

difficulty tolerating any of the dilating agents, but by trial and error a suitable one can usually be found.

Calcium channel antagonists selectively block the movement of calcium ions, so influx of calcium into the cells is reduced and thus smooth muscle contractility is decreased. Some of these agents also have alpha-adrenoreceptor blocking activity, a beneficial effect on red blood cell deformability, an antiaggregating action on platelets, and an ability to inhibit platelet synthesis of thromboxane A2, a vasoconstrictor and platelet activator. They have been shown to be particularly effective for inhibiting vascular responses evoked by alpha-adrenoreceptor activity. These receptors are predominately activated during reflex sympathetic stimulation from body cooling.[3, 4] These agents should not be given to subjects with moderate or severe left ventricular systolic dysfunction, and only cautiously with mild myocardial depression.[5]

The calcium entry blockers differ in their cardiac and peripheral activity, with felodipine (plendil) and nifedipine (Adalat; Apo-Nifed; Novonifedin; Procardia) having the most potent peripheral vasodilator action. A dose of 10 to 20 mg four times a day is required. Side effects (transient hypotension, dizziness, flushing, headache, edema) may be reduced by commencing therapy with a small dose. Diltiazem HCL (Apo-diltiaz, Cardizem, Tilazem) is an alternative. Verapamil HCL (Isoptin, Calan, Cordilox, Dilacoran, Manidon, Vasolan) seems to be less effective.

Alternative peripheral vasodilator drugs that may be beneficial include prazosin HCL (Minipress and Hypovase), which directly relaxes smooth muscle and to some extent interferes with peripheral sympathetic function, cyclandelate (Cyclospasmol), tolazoline HCL (Priscoline), nicotinyl alcohol tartrate (Roniacol Supraspan), raubasine (Hydrosarpan-Fort), and inositol niacinate (Linodil), which may in addition relieve muscle cramp, a troublesome symptom. Thymoxamine, an alpha-adrenoreceptor antagonist blocks vasoconstriction in the skin while maintaining overall vascular resistance.[6]

The necessity for drug therapy increases with the severity of Raynaud's phenomenon. The correct agent will successfully prevent blanching attacks in 50–80 percent of workers.[7]

Blood Rheology

Another group of drugs that may be useful are those that inhibit thromboxane synthetase or promote antiplatelet vasodilator effects.[8] These include dazoxiben, dipyridamole (Asasantine, Persantine), pentoxifylline (Trental) and the prostanoids—prostaglandin E1 (Alprostadil, Prostin VR, Minprog) or its analogues. Given orally, or by intravenous infusion, they reduce platelet adhesiveness (deaggregation), improve the flexibility of red blood cells, and cause generalised vasodilation.[9-12] This line of treatment has been shown to be effective in patients with severe symptoms where digits are at risk from tissue necrosis.

Nitrates such as isosorbide dinitrate (Cedocard-SR, Coradur, Coronex, Isordil, Norosorbide, Apo-ISDN) release nitric oxide in vivo, and when used in combination with prostaglandin E1, synergize and reduce platelet deposition and increase platelet survival time.[13]

In advanced cases when other methods have failed, and if there is an associated scleroderma, fibrinolytic activity enhancing agents such as Stanozolol (Winstrol; stromba) are effective.[14, 15]

Blood Viscosity

Plasmapheresis or plasma exchange therapy has been recorded as being of value[16, 17] for severe cases with digital ulcers. There are risks associated with the use of blood products, and any improvement induced by the treatment occurs by an unknown mechanism.

Biofeedback

For some cases, biofeedback techniques have been advocated.[18] The main objective is to overcome emotional stress. Adherents to this technique postulate that stress is wholly sufficient to induce vasospastic episodes. They postulate that corrective conditioning produces blood vessel musculature responses, reduced HAVS attacks, and raised finger temperatures may follow from training sessions, usually more than six. To be successful subjects require visual recognition (impact) of the irregularities to be overcome (for example, blood flow reduction, cold finger). Researchers in this area[19, 20] are convinced that biofeedback is an effective, holistic, symptomatic treatment. The number of patients treated to date is small and the conclusions are not as yet convincing; however, using combination techniques (that is, biofeedback with hypnosis, relaxation training, and autogenic suggestion) a greater success rate is claimed.

Surgery and Physiotherapy

Surgical intervention for HAVS in the form of cervical sympathectomy or stellate ganglion block to improve peripheral circulation, or release of nerve entrapment for associated carpal tunnel syndrome, (CTS) although frequently used in the past, has given disappointing results. Hence surgery is used less frequently today, usually as a last resort in the most severe cases. In a follow-up study of 41 men treated surgically for associated CTS it was concluded that surgery reduced but did not eliminate all symptoms in all cases, and that high exposure to vibration may result in poorer recovery.[21] If the subject has to continue HAV exposure on economic grounds, surgery may be justified. In 10 percent to 20 percent of cases results are unsatisfactory.

The advocates of physical therapy treatments reported in the literature fail to support their findings with age/sex matched controls. Furthermore the evaluation of the treatment by self-assessment is purely subjective and has not been confirmed by recognized objective tests. In many of the surveys, neuroticism in the study subjects has been as high as 33 percent.[22]

Depending on the severity of the condition the preferred treatment of most patients is generally a combination of vasodilator and symptomatic analgesic drugs. In some patients it may be necessary to provide connective tissue massage and physical therapy for the musculoskeletal symptoms.[23-25] We should aim at providing patients with as clear an understanding of their disease as possible and use the drugs and therapy available with circumspection, remembering that treatment is likely to be lifelong. Decisions should be made with, rather than for, the patient, making it possible to share disappointment at failure and satisfaction when treatment is effective.[26]

PREVENTION AND MANAGEMENT

For the prevention of finger blanching, cold exposure should be avoided as far as possible. Wearing warm dry clothes, to maintain a raised central body core temperature, is also a most useful and important aid. Muffs are preferable to gloves, and inserts may be necessary. Electrically heated gloves are available for severe cases. The feet should also be protected by thick socks and fur-lined boots when temperatures are extreme. Hand and foot warmers can be used to advantage. Tobacco smoking should be avoided.

Control and elimination of HAVS from the workplace is multifactorial and all elements have to be identified and controlled or eliminated to solve the problem.[27] The NIOSH criteria document[28] in the section on worker protection addresses the main items. Because the development of HAVS is dose-related, effective control procedures should be directed primarily to reducing the intensity (acceleration) of the vibration, reducing the exposure duration, identifying the early signs and symptoms, and identifying vibration-sensitive individuals. Control strategies should include exposure monitoring to assess the risk, engineering controls to avoid or reduce HAV exposure, work practices to reduce exposure, ergonomic considerations to reduce muscular activity and strain, protective clothing and equipment to attenuate vibration and avoid cold exposure, worker monitoring to ensure good practice, and medical monitoring to identify any early manifestations of HAVS.

Identification of the hazard and its severity by vibration measurement, and reduction at the source of transmission are discussed in Chapter 11. The ergonomic considerations, particularly in respect of tool weight, tool grip, angle of operation, work speed, et cetera, are addressed in Chapters 8 and 11. In addition, practical and acceptable work practices need to be implemented to reduce the health impact of using vibrating tools. This may mean reducing the exposure time during the day, week, month, and year with the introduction of exposure/nonexposure cycles by job rotation or rest periods.[29]

Protective clothing and equipment should aim to reduce transmission of vibration energy to the hand and protect the hands from exposure to cold and trauma. Vibration-damping materials are now available for incorporation into gloves and mittens. They have to provide adequate damping with minimal thickness so that the dexterity required for safe and efficient tool operation will not be reduced. Such materials must attenuate vibration over the damaging frequency range from 30 to 300 Hz. Present materials attenuate high-frequency vibration, but at levels below 500 Hz, attenuation is minimal. In some instances the use of gloves has increased the vibration through resonance of the absorbent material used in glove manufacture (see chapters 9 and 11).

Worker training is critical in order that they may be alerted to the hazard, the need to service their hand tools regularly in order to minimize the vibration, to grip the tools as lightly as possible within the bounds of safety, use the protective clothing equipment, attend for medical surveillance, and to report all signs and symptoms of HAVS as soon as they develop.

Medical surveillance, in addition to routine monitoring, should provide health education. The health counselling should include alerting workers to the nature of the disease and to avoid smoking. The clinical evaluation at the preplacement and periodic examinations should include some or all of the items discussed in Chapter 5. The frequency of the periodic examination will be determined by the nature of the risk and the severity of the symptoms and signs (see Chapter 3). Advice from the clinician whether the worker should continue to be exposed to vibration, having developed signs and symptoms, will depend on the jurisdiction and the legal practice of the country, and the company's medical policy. However, it has been established that at stage 2, without further HAV exposure, recovery from all the symptoms and signs is possible. It is preferable for workers to change their occupation, if this is feasible, at this stage. If not, administrative controls should be adopted to reduce the exposure dose, and drug therapy may be necessary.

SUMMARY

The treatment of HAVS patients will depend on the stage. Mild cases should avoid cold exposure as much as possible and be encouraged to restore circulation to blanched fingers by swinging the arms. At stage 2 vascular (Stockholm) further HAV exposure should be avoided if possible, so that recovery with loss of symptoms and signs may occur. Therapy with a calcium ion inhibitor, such as felodipine, should be prescribed for workers with symptoms. Surgical intervention for both HAVS and for associated CTS should be avoided as far as possible.

Notes

1. Matoba, T. and Sakurai, T. "Treatments for Vibration Disease." *Scand. J. Work. Environ. Health* 1986; 12: 259-261.
2. Matoba, T. and Kuwahara H. "Treatment for Hand-Arm Vibration Disease in Japan." *Karume Med. J.* 1990; 37:123-126.
3. Coffman, J. D. "Treatment." In. Coffman, J. D., ed. *Raynaud's Phenomenon.* New York: Oxford University Press, 1989: 127-166.
4. Roath, S. "Managing Raynaud's Phenomenon." *BMJ* 1986; 293:88-89.
5. Anonymous. "Calcium Antagonist Caution" (Editorial). *Lancet* 1991; 337:885-886.
6. Lindblad, L. E., and Ekenvall, L. "Alpha 2-Adrenoceptor Inhibition in Patients With Vibration White Fingers." *Kurume Med. J.* 1990; 37:95-99.
7. Matoba and Sakurai, "Treatments for Vibration Disease."
8. Roath, "Managing Raynaud's Phenomenon."
9. Ibid.
10. Cooke, E. D., and Nicolaides, A. N. "Raynaud's Syndrome." *BMJ* 1990; 300:553-555.
11. Vane, J. R. "Prostacyclin in Health and Disease." Lilly Lecture, 1981. *Royal Coll. Phys. Edin. Publ. No. 58,* 1982.
12. Dowd, P. M.; Martin, M. F. R.; Cooke, E. D.; Bow-cock, S. A.; Jones, R.; Dieppe, P. A.; Kirby, J. D. "Treatment of Raynaud's Phenomenon by Intravenous Infusion of Prostacyclin (PGI$_2$)." *Brit. J. Dermatology* 1982; 106:81-89.
13. Sinzinger, H.; Fitscha, P.; O'Grady, J.; Rauscha, F.; Rogatti, W.; Vane, J. R. "Synergistic Effect of Prostaglandin E1 and Isosorbide Dinitrate in Peripheral Vascular Disease." *Lancet* 1990; 335:627-628.
14. Jarrett, P. E. M.; Morland, M.; Browse, N. L. "Treatment of Raynaud's Phenomenon by Fibrinolytic Enhancement." *BMJ* 1978; 2:523-525.
15. Nasu, Y. "Defibrinogating Therapy for Peripheral Circulatory Disturbance in Patients With Vibration Syndrome." *Scand. J. Work. Environ. Health* 1986; 12:272-276.
16. Roath, "Managing Raynaud's Phenomenon."
17. Dodds, A. J.; O'Reilly, M. J. G.; Yates, C. P. "Haemorrheological Response to Plasma Exchange in Raynaud's Syndrome." *BMJ* 1979; 2:1186-1187.
18. Yocum, D. E.; Hodes, R.; Sundstrom, W. R.; Cleeland, C. S. "Use of Biofeedback Training in Treatment of Raynaud's Disease and Phenomenon." *J. Rheumatol.* 1985; 12:90-93.
19. Ibid.
20. Sappington, J. T.; Fiorito, E. M.; Brehony, K. A. "Biofeedback as Therapy in Raynaud's Phenomenon." *Biofeedback and Self-Regulation* 1979; 4(2):155-168.
21. Hagberg, M.; Nystrom, A.; Zetterlund, B. "Recovery From Symptoms After Carpal Tunnel Syndrome Surgery in Males in Relation to Vibration Exposure." *J. Hand Surg.* 1991; 16A:66-71.
22. Matoba and Sakurai, "Treatments for Vibration Disease."
23. Matoba and Kuwahara, "Treatment for Hand-Arm Vibration."
24. Färkkilä, M., and Pyykkö, I. "Treatment of Vibration Syndrome in Finland." *Kurume Med. J.* 1990; 37:127-128.
25. Bovenzi, M. and Zadini, A. "Treatment of the Hand-Arm Vibration Syndrome in Italy." *Kurume Med. J.* 1990; 37:129-130.
26. Cooke and Nicolaides, "Raynaud's Syndrome."

27. Wasserman, D. E. "The Control and Elimination of Vibration in the Workplace." In: Wasserman, D. E., ed. *Human Aspects of Occupational Vibration*. New York: Elsevier, 1987: 145-157.
28. "Criteria for a Recommend Standard. Occupational Exposure to Hand-Arm Vibration." 1989. DHHS (NIOSH) publication No. 89-106.
29. Saito, K. "Prevention of the Hand-Arm Vibration Syndrome." *Scand. J. Work. Environ. Health* 1987; 13:301-304.

7

Epidemiology of Hand-Arm Vibration Syndrome

V. J. Behrens, P. L. Pelmear

Raynaud's phenomenon of occupational origin has been recognized since 1911 when Loriga in Rome[1] reported "dead fingers" among the Italian miners who used pneumatic tools. Such tools had been introduced into the French mines in 1839 and were being extensively used by 1890.

In the United States pneumatic tools were first introduced into the limestone quarries of Bedford, Indiana, about 1896. The health hazards associated with their use, both pulmonary and neurological, were noted subsequently by Leake.[2] This lead to an investigation in 1917–1918 by the U.S. Bureau of Labor under the direction of Dr. Alice Hamilton, with the full support of the Journeyman Stone Cutters Association.[3] Dr. Hamilton and her colleagues, Drs. Cary, Cottingham, and Rothstein examined 166 workers using pneumatic impact hammers to cut and dress stone. Ninety percent of the limestone cutters in Bedford, Indiana; 86 percent of the granite cutters in Vermont, Massachusetts; and 56 percent of the marble workers in Vermont, Long Island City, and Baltimore had experienced Raynaud's phenomenon. Dr. Hamilton's classical description of Raynaud's phenomenon has not been surpassed in the subsequent literature. Many years elapsed before stone cutters in Europe were reported to be similarly affected.[4]

First reports of hand-arm vibration syndrome (HAVS) in workers exposed to hand-arm vibration (HAV) from specific tools and work situations have continued since then.

1911 **Compressed air tools** in French mines. Ref: Loriga, G. "Pneumatic Tools." Quoted by Teleky, L. *Occup. Health Sup. ILO* 1938:1–12.

1918 **Compressed air tools,** Indiana lime stone quarries. Ref: Hamilton, A. "A Study of Spastic Anaemia in the Hands of Stonecutters." Bulletin 236. U.S. Bureau Labor Stat. 1918; 19:53–66.

1931 **Grinding wheels** (compressed air). Ref: Seyring, M. "Maladies From Work With Compressed Air Tools." *Bull Hyg.* 1931; 6:25.

1940 **Cutlery grinding.** Ref: Cummins, R. C. "'Dead hand': A Lesion Produced by Rapid Vibration." *Irish. J. Med. Sci.* 1940; 171-175.

1945 **Pneumatic drills** (airplane manufacturing). Ref: Gurdjian, E. S.; and Walker, L. W. "Traumatic Vasospastic Disease of the Hand (White Fingers). *JAMA* 1945; 129:668-672.

1945 **Fettlers, riveters, and caulkers.** Ref: Hunter, D.; McLaughlin, A. I. G.; Perry, K. M. A. "Clinical Effects of the Use of Pneumatic Tools." *Brit. J. Ind. Med.* 1945; 2:10-16.

1945 **Polishing** (electrically driven). Ref: Telford, E. D.; McCann, M. B.; MacCormack, D. H. "Dead Hand" in Users of Vibrating Tools. *Lancet* 1945; 2:359-360.

1962 **Jackleg hammers and stoper drills.** Ref: Williams, N. and Riegert, A. L. "Raynaud's Phenomenon of Occupational Origin in Uranium Miners." In: Proceedings of the 13th International Congress on Occupational Health. New York. 1962: 819-825.

1964 **Chain saws** (Tasmania). Ref: Grounds, M. D. "Raynaud's Phenomenon in Users of Chain Saws." *Med. J. Aust* 1964; 1:270-272.

1966 **Chain saws** (Japan). Ref: Muira, T; Kimura, K; Tominga, Y; Kimotsuki, K. "On the Raynaud's Phenomenon of Occupational Origin due to Vibrating Tool—It's Incidence in Japan." *Report of the Institute for Science and Labour.* 1966; 65:1-11.

1968 **Chain saws** (Sweden). Ref: Axelson, S. "Analysis of Vibration in Power Saws." No.59, Skogshogskolan, Royal College of Forestry Monograph, Stockholm. 1968.

1971 **Chain saws** (U.K.). Ref: Taylor, W.; Pearson, J.; Kell, R. L.; Keighley, G. D. "Vibration Syndrome in Forestry Commission Chain Saw Operators." *Brit. J. Ind. Med.* 1971; 28:83-89.

1972 **Chain saws** (Norway). Ref: Hellstrom, B.; and Andersen, K. L. "Vibration Injuries in Norwegian Forest Workers." *Brit. J. Ind. Med.* 1972; 29:255-263.

1979 **Brush Cutters** (Japan). Ref: Futatsuku, M. "A Study on the Vibration Hazards due to Using Brush Cutters." *Jpn. J. Health* 1979; 21:269-273.

1982 **Motorcycle Speedway Riders** (U.K.). Ref: Bentley, S; O'Conner, D. E.; Lord, P.; Edmonds, O. P. "Vibration White Finger in Motorcycle Speedway Riders." In: Brammer, A. J. and Taylor, W, eds. *Vibration Effects on the Hand and Arm in Industry.* New York: John Wiley & Sons, 1982:189-192.

The number at risk in the United States in 1974 was estimated to be 1.25 million (see Table 7-1)[5] and in 1983 it was nearer 1.5 million. The United States however was lulled into a false state of security by the report of Pecora et al[6] in 1960. As investigators with the public health service, they sent letters of inquiry to 50

TABLE 7-1   Workers Potentially Exposed to Hand-Arm Vibration

Number of Workers	Industry	Type of Tool
500,000	Construction	Hand tools
200,000	Farming	Gasoline chain saws
14,000	Metal working	Hand tools
54,000	Steel	Furnace cleaning using powered hand tools
30,000	Lumber and wood	Gasoline chain saws
34,000	Furniture manufacturing	Hand tools
100,000	Mining	Pneumatic drills
250,000	Truck and auto manufacturing	Hand tools
64,000	Foundries	Hand tools

Total 1,246,000

Ref: "Vibration Syndrome." Current Intelligence Bulletin 38. 1983 DHHS (NIOSH) Publication No. 83-110.

American states, county, and city industrial agencies to assess the numbers of persons exposed to vibratory tools and the numbers reporting disease from sustained use. Discussions were held with industrial physicians and 11 large plants were visited. No cases of Raynaud's phenomenon of occupational origin were found and the authors stated "the impression from industry is that Raynaud's phenomenon of occupational origin from vibration from hand tools is practically nonexistent since no cases had been reported in the last ten years, and no compensation claim for this disease had been paid." They concluded that vibration syndrome "may become an uncommon occupational disease approaching extinction in this country." This conclusion was shown to be wrong by the subsequent NIOSH 1981 study by Wasserman et al.[7]

In Great Britain, in the early 70s, the Department of Health and Social Security (DHSS) in connection with an investigation by the Industrial Injuries Advisory Council into the vibration syndrome supported two major studies: one by Stewart and Goda[8] and another by Taylor and Pelmear.[9] From an investigation carried out in Great Britain by the Health and Safety Executive (HSE), between 1984 and 1986 in selected manufacturing sectors, it was estimated that approximately 130,000 workers were exposed to HAV for relatively long periods, and in the construction industry on any working day about 22,000 workers were exposed to HAV all day.[10, 11] The number of workers exposed by industry and type of tool is given in Figures 7-1 and 7-2.

To appreciate the risk to workers and to follow how the knowledge base has developed over the years, it is preferable to review the epidemiological reports by association with the tool used and/or the work situation.

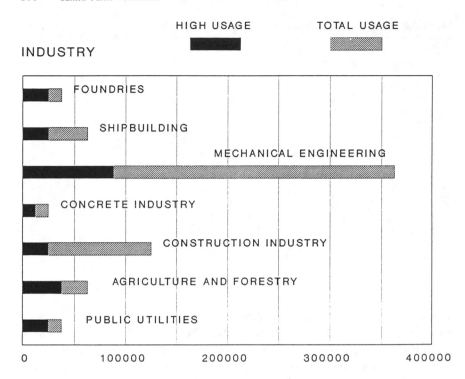

NUMBER OF WORKERS EXPOSED

FIGURE 7-1.   Manual Workeers Exposed to Hand-Arm Vibration, HSE Survey 1987.   *Source:* Bednall, A.W. "Hand-Arm Vibration in Great Britian." In: Proceedings of the Fifth International Conference on Low Frequency Noise and Vibration. Oxford: Multi-Science Publishing Co., 1989: 13–20.

PNEUMATIC TOOLS

Grinding as a cause of Raynaud's phenomenon was first reported by Seyring in 1931.[12] She made a special investigation of cleaners of castings and analogus processes, and found that the liability to this condition increases with the years exposed; 4 percent suffering within two years; 48 percent within two to three years; 55 percent within ten years; and 61 percent after ten years. It was most prevalent among those cleaners who used their air drills on very hard resisting material. Cummins[13] reported the case of a worker developing symptoms after three months exposure to work on cutlery grinding.

The first report of HAVS in pneumatic drill users in airplane manufacturing was by Gurdjian and Walker in 1945.[14] Six women engaged in aircraft construction were

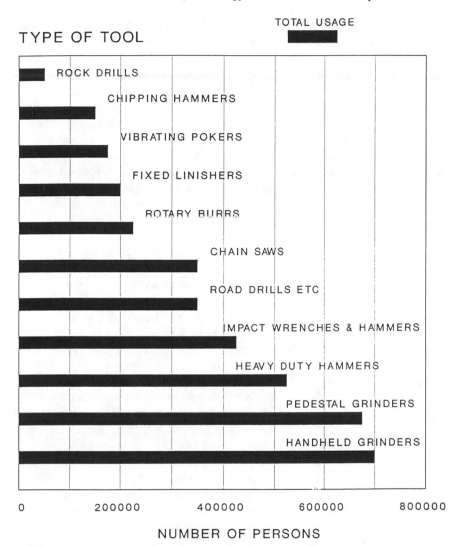

FIGURE 7-2.   Ranking of Tools in the Term of Number of People Using Them.

affected, the latent interval being 10–11 months. Reports on other drill users followed.[15, 16] Hunter et al.[17] examining 286 pneumatic tool workers in various trades, found the prevalence to be 71 percent in fettlers, 74 percent in riveters and 82 percent in caulkers. The latent period was two to five years. Similar findings were reported by Magos and Okos[18] in the Hungarian iron, steel, and engineering industry. In addition to compressed-air driven fettling tools, electrically driven fettling tools were also found to cause HAVS.[19, 20]

Agate and co-workers,[22-24] in the period 1947–1949, reported high prevalence rates (over 86 percent) in foundry grinders. The mean latent interval was two years.

Caulkers and paint chippers in shipyards are also at risk. Oliver et al.,[25] in the U.K. dockyards, found a prevalence of 75 percent among caulkers and 18 percent in paint chippers. Bovenzi et al.,[26] in 1980, examined 169 caulkers employed at a shipyard and found that 78.7 percent experienced paresthesia in their hands, 31.3 percent Raynaud's phenomenon, 31.3 percent with cysts of the carpal bones, 20.1 percent with radiological oestoarthritis of wrists and shoulders, and 10 percent with olecranon exostoses. NIOSH conducted surveys in two foundries and one shipyard in the United States and collected data on 385 workers exposed to vibration.[27] The prevalence of HAVS in the exposed group was 47 percent at the foundries and 19 percent at the shipyard. None of the workers in the control group had Raynaud's phenomenon. The median latent interval was 1.4 years among foundry workers and 16.5 years among shipyard workers. The severity of HAVS increased significantly in proportion to the number of years that the foundry and shipyard workers used the chipping hammers. Behrens et al.,[28] in 1984 subsequently noted that the prevalence was greater among incentive workers than among the hourly paid. Jepson,[29] in 1954, investigating 34 patients with HAVS, observed that it was common for the condition to be more severe in fingers to which most vibration was transmitted.

In the early 1960s HAVS was reported in hard-rock miners using jackleg hammers and stoper drills in Canada.[30-32] Subsequently reports came from Europe,[33-35] Japan,[36, 37] and Korea,[38] together with further reports from Canada[39-44] and America.[45] The prevalence rates ranged from 12.5–50 percent and the median latent intervals from 4.5–17 years.

The stonecutters of Bedford, Indiana, were revisited in 1978 by Taylor et al.[46] The Alice Hamilton investigation found a prevalence of 89 percent in 1918 and the prevalence was still 80 percent in 1978. Bovenzi et al.,[47] in 1988, surveyed a similar group of stone drillers and stonecutters/chippers working in the Rapolano travertine quarries in Tuscany, Italy. The prevalence of HAVS was 35.5 percent with a mean latent interval of ten years.

Musson et al.,[48] in 1989, in a questionnaire survey of 445 workers using chipping hammers, jack hammers, and road breakers in small companies throughout the Netherlands had a response rate of 38 percent. From this data they established a prevalence of 17 percent for HAVS, and back pain showed an increase in prevalence with increasing total time exposed to vibration. But Walker et al.,[49] in 1985, interviewing a similar group of workers in the United Kingdom, gas industry, found that the prevalence of HAVS in the group exposed to vibration at work was 9.6 percent compared with 9.5 percent in the control group. That no particular problem was found may have been due to the relatively short exposures to vibration experienced by the operators over a long period extending beyond 30 years (that is, intermittent vibration exposure).

Nilsson et al.,[50] in 1989, studied 89 platers who were exposed to HAV from grinders and die grinders in Sweden. The prevalence was 42 percent and the mean latent interval was 9.8 years.

Pedestal grinders using zirconia (70 percent aluminum oxide and 30 percent zirconium oxide) wheels, as opposed to silicon carbide or carborundum wheels, are particularly at risk. Pelmear et al.,[51] in a group of 26 pedestal grinders, found that the prevalence of HAVS was 96 percent with a mean latent interval of 1.8 years. This high risk was confirmed subsequently by Starck et al.[52] in a similar group of pedestal grinders in Finland. The mean latent interval there was 10.3 months. It was concluded that some feature, such as the impulsive percussive character of the vibration, contributed to the high risk and short latent interval.

CHAIN SAWS

The chain saw was first introduced to timber fellers in Germany before the Second World War, and in Sweden in ever increasing numbers in the early 1950s. The chain saw powered by a small petrol driven motor is now widely used for the forest operations of felling, snedding, and crosscutting in all timber-growing countries.

It became apparent that the operators were at risk of Raynaud's phenomenon in 1964 when Grounds[53] found 20 of 22 men affected in the district of Maydena, Tasmania. The latent interval was as short as one year. The climate in Maydena (temperatures 33°–72°F) is cold by Australian standards. Reports from Japan and Sweden followed.[54-56] Barnes et al.[57] were asked by the New South Wales State Forestry Commission to investigate the incidence among timber workers on the north coast of New South Wales. Of the 80 chain saw operators examined, 50 percent were affected. The latent interval varied from one to ten years. None of the workers at the time of the interview were contemplating giving up the work, and they considered the condition more of an annoyance than a disability. The authors were of the opinion that vibration disease at least in the warmer parts of Australia, presents apparently little difficulty, which may have explained why so few patients consulted a doctor even though the condition was relatively common.

An investigation by the Forestry Commission of Great Britain and the Department of Social and Occupational Medicine at the University of Dundee was reported in 1971 by Taylor et al.[58,59] A questionnaire was put to 800 random selected employees and 732 responded (97 percent). Of the 142 chain saw operators, 44 percent had Raynaud's phenomenon compared with 18 percent in the nonusers. An increase in prevalence with the years of chain saw usage was found, starting at around two years with a marked increase (73 percent) at over eight years. Hellstrom and Andersen,[60] in 1972, in a similar study in Norway reported a prevalence of 47 percent in chain saw operators, 14 percent in nonuser forestry workers, and 9 percent in indoor workers among forestry workers in three areas of east Norway. The mean latent interval was eight years. Subsequently Taylor et al.[61] reported the results of examinations on 46 chain saw operators who had been surveyed annually for 11 years. The prevalence of vibration white finger (VWF) in this population group when first seen was 85 percent, but after the introduction of antivibration saws the prevalence rate declined to 30 percent. The prevalence rate in controls was 6 percent.

The reported prevalence rates in Canadian chain saw users was 30.5 percent and 8.7 percent among nonusers,[62] and in Finnish lumberjacks 40 percent.[63]

Antivibration saws were introduced in the early 70s, and follow-up studies attempted to evaluate their benefit, if any. Futatsuka and Ueno[64-66] monitored 1,456 workers in the national forests of Western Japan over the period 1956-1980. Although prevalence by duration of exposure in each cohort increased, there was an overall decrease in prevalence and incidence over time, due to reduced exposure time to vibration as well as a reduction in the level. Pyykkö et al.,[67,68] in a follow-up study of Finnish forestry workers during the period 1972-1983 likewise noted a reduction in prevalence of HAVS from 40 percent among the workers in 1972 to 5 percent in 1983. However Brubaker et al.[69,70] monitoring coastal fellers in British Columbia, Canada, noted a prevalence of 51 percent in 1979-1980, which did not differ significantly from a prevalence of 53 percent in 1984-1985. Reported recovery and improvement in the group with symptoms in 1979-1980 was counter balanced by a significant 30 percent onset of new symptoms among fellers who were asymptomatic in 1979-1980. Six of the eight fellers reporting new symptoms were exposed only to antivibration saws.

Pelnar et al.,[71] in a survey of 566 forestry workers in Quebec and Ontario, Canada, noted a prevalence rate of 27.9 percent.

Miyashita et al.,[72] in 1983, suggested total operating time (TOT) as an index of vibration dose. The total chain saw operating time was calculated by using the following equation: chain saw operating hours/day × days/year × years. Two hundred and sixty-six chain saw operators were classified into four groups and 46 forestry workers not using chain saws were used as controls. In the group with under 2,000 hours experience (15 percent), symptoms were generally confined to tingling, numbness, or pain; with 2,000-5,000 hours (28 percent) peripheral nerve and circulatory disturbances, including Raynaud's phenomenon, and muscle and general body conditions were present to some degree; with 5,000-8,000 hours (19 percent) functional changes were noted; while with over 8,000 hours (38 percent) about half the operators suffered severely from functional or organic changes due to vibration.

Futatsuka et al.[73] used principal component analysis to determine the interrelationships between subjective symptoms experienced by workers using various types of vibrating tools, (that is, brush saws, rock drills, chipping hammers, or chain saws) and a control group of clerks and farmers. The prevalence rates of complaints in the subject groups were noted and the subjects were matched for age. From a wide variety of symptoms a principal component related to peripheral nerves, to muscle and joints, and a component for peripheral circulation were extracted. The complaints of the rock drillers reflected a peripheral circulatory factor whereas those of the chain saw operators and the chipping hammer operators presented a complex factor of nerves, muscles, and joints.

OTHER SOURCES

Speedway and dirt-track racing are popular sports in many countries. The engines are rigidly bolted to the frame, normally there is no gear box or brakes, and the handle bar is bolted to the steering head. In a survey of riders competing in the British speedway racing league, Bentley et al.[74] reported a very high prevalence of HAVS (94 percent, id est, 30 of 32 riders being affected), with a latent interval of five years.

Brush saws are hand-held, vibrating power tools used primarily in forestry and agriculture, for grass cutting, and by workmen engaged in maintainence of rural parks and roadsides. In Japanese studies[75-78] the prevalence of HAVS among brush saw operators seems to be lower than that observed in other forestry workers such as chain saw users. However the occurrence of sensorineural and musculoskeletal disorders is reported to be higher.[79] Bovenzi et al.[80] conducted an experimental study of the physiological effects of brush saw operation on eight professional agricultural workers. A variety of tests were used and they confirmed that the risk of HAVS among brush saw users was low. A particularly high-risk occupation group were swaging operators who handled copper tubes. The swaging machine reduced the diameter at the end of the tubes to form a solid fulcrum. The operators had to hold the tube very tightly during this operation. Taylor et al.[81] found that they had a latent interval of six months to nine months (mean 0.6 years).

HAVS REVERSIBILITY

Until the 1950s, clinicians held the view that the signs and symptoms of HAVS were irreversible. Evidence that improvement or reversal of the vascular symptoms could occur on withdrawing the worker from vibration exposure first came from Stewart and Goda[81] in 1970, and Riddle and Taylor,[83] Hursch[84] and Pyykkö et al.[45] from surveys in 1982. During the 1990s, worldwide surveys led to the conclusion that the observed VWF prevalence improvement was due to the introduction of antivibration saws reducing the vibration intensity and administrative controls that curtailed the saw usage time. It was presumed that reducing the vibration dosage decreased the abnormal reactivity of the peripheral vessels, with a regression of vessel wall structural damage. Later, in 1985, Futatsuka et al.[86] showed that the percentage improvement depended on the severity at the time the vibration exposure ceased, that the reversibility was influenced by age (increasing age less improvement), and that the "numbness" of hands appeared to be more resistant to reversibility. Recent surveys by Ekenvall and Carlsson[87] in 1987, and by Olsen and Nielsen[88] in 1988, both using objective tests (finger systolic pressure and cold-water immersion tests) to evaluate improvement, confirmed the trend in VWF reversal. The surveys did not provide data on which the rate and degree of improvement could be precisely established. The reason for this absence of hard data is due to the number of confounding variables:

a. The improvement is largely dependent on the subjects own assessment of his or her disability, including recall.
b. Established cases of VWF learning to adapt by avoiding cold environments and retaining central body core temperature.
c. The disability is recognized by the subject, so stress and worry over circulation in the hands is reduced.

In the surveys reported, many have relied purely on the subjective history. There is as yet no hard data available based on internationally approved objective tests together with their normative data. That there is partial recovery in advanced cases (stage 2 and 3, under age 40 years) has been shown by James and Galloway[89] who showed collateral vessel development to bypass digital arteries blocked by thrombus and/or by intima and medial coat hyperplasia. The evidence for reversibility of the vascular component of HAVS on removal of the vibration stimulus may be summarized as follows:

a. In a small proportion of stage 1V and early stage 2V (Stockholm) cases the vascular symptoms will improve and, in some cases, disappear on removal from exposure (that is, there is positive evidence of reversibility).
b. In the more severe cases at stages 2V and 3V (Stockholm) recovery is unlikely. There is positive evidence that the more severe the case, the longer will be the reversal time.
c. There is some evidence in respect of the influence of age on workers—the older the impaired worker the longer the reversal time. However the older worker (over 40 years) may not recover due to the onset of arteriosclerosis.
d. Recent evidence from clinicians with instrumentation for measuring the sensorineural component of HAVS is that the sensory component is slower to reverse, if indeed there is any measurable recovery.

CONCLUSION

It is apparent from these epidemiological studies that HAVS is a twentieth century disease. Almost any hand-held vibrating tool will affect the vascular, sensorineural, and musculoskeletal structures of the upper limbs of workers. The critical factor is vibration dose, which is a product of vibration level and exposure time. There is a positive correlation between exposure time and the severity of HAVS.

Some of the studies have found workers recovering from HAVS after discontinuing exposure, and others have been able to report some recovery following the use of antivibration chain saws. In addition, the use of antivibration chain saws has prolonged the latent interval (that is, the time between first exposure and the development of Raynaud's phenomenon).

The majority of the studies reviewed have estimated risk from prevalence and incidence rates. This is unsatisfactory since worker populations are notoriously mobile so the prevalence will vary from one month to another. Epidemiologists have found that latent intervals are a much better indicator of hazard and therefore should be used when evaluating the risk in any work situation. The correlation of "latent interval" and vibration dosage has been established in many studies.

Wasserman and Taylor[90] have drawn attention to some of the problems and issues in HAVS epidemiological studies. Some of the early studies did not consider all the factors. The determination of the risk to populations of workers requires the evaluation of a number of factors, including variation in individual exposures, the turnover rate, the reasons for leaving, and the reason for survivors being unaffected. Bias must be avoided in the collection and interpretation of data, and the study design should permit the identification and evaluation of modifiers and confounders such as the influence of wearing gloves, vibration-free rest periods, work practices, tool condition, smoking, age, and core body temperatures. For the proper epidemiological evaluation of HAVS a team of physicians, epidemiologists, engineers, and scientists is required. This must be a team effort, and it is a unique challenge for today's researchers representing many disciplines.

To date most of the studies have evaluated risk using "weighted" vibration measurements as opposed to "unweighted." Recommended safety standards using weighted data are now being questioned.[91-94] The standards appear to be less protective where there is a significant high-frequency component in the vibration source spectra. Consequently NIOSH, in 1989, called for further studies with both "weighted" and "unweighted" vibration measurements.[95] There is an urgent need for such data using unweighted measurements in epidemiological studies.

SUMMARY

Workers were first exposed to HAV from pneumatic tools in 1839 and the first report of Raynaud's phenomenon of occupational origin from their use was in 1911. As pneumatic tools became more widely used, epidemiological reports by association with tool used and/or work situation (for example, quarrying, mining, foundries, ship and aircraft manufacturer) appeared with increasing frequency in the medical literature.

Chain saws came into common use in the 1950s and epidemiological reports of HAVS in forestry workers in many parts of the world started to appear in the 1960s. It is apparent from these epidemiological studies that HAVS is a twentieth century disease, and that almost any hand-held vibratory tool will affect the vascular, sensorineural, and musculoskeletal structures of the limbs. The critical factor is vibration dose, which is a product of vibration level and exposure time. There is always a latent interval between first exposure and the onset of Raynaud's phenomenon. In general the greater the risk the shorter the interval. There is a positive correlation between exposure time and the severity of HAVS. The use of antivibration devices on tools, particularly chains saws, have extended the latent intervals.

Most of the epidemiological studies have evaluated risk using "weighted" vibration measurements. The safety standards based on this data are now being increasingly questioned.

Notes

1. Loriga, G. "Il Lavoro Con i Martelli Pneumatici." *Boll Inspett Lavoro* 1911; 2:35–60.
2. Leake, J. P. "Health Hazards From the Use of the Air Hammer in Cutting Indiana Limestone." *Ind. Accident Hyg. Series*, Bulletin 236, No. 19. U.S. Dept. of Labor, Bureau of Labor Statistics 1918:100–113.
3. Hamilton, A. "A Study of Spastic Anaemia in the Hands of Stonecutters."*Ind. Accident Hyg. Services*, Bulletin 236, No. 19. U.S. Dept. of Labor, Bureau of Labor Statistics 1918:53–66.
4. Hardgrove, M. A. F. and Barker, N. W. "Pneumatic Hammer Disease: A Vasospastic Disturbance of the Hands in Stonecutters." *Proc. Staff Meeting*, Mayo Clinic 1933; 8:345–349.
5. *Vibration Syndrome.* 1983. DHHS (NIOSH) Publication No. 83-110.
6. Percora, L. J. "Survey of Current Status of Raynaud's Phenomenon of Occupational Origin." *J. Amer. Ind. Hyg. Assoc.* 1960:21–80.
7. Wasserman, D. E.; Taylor, W. Behrens, V.; Samueloff, S.; Reynolds, D. "Vibration White Finger Disease in U.S. Workers Using Pneumatic Chipping and Grinding Hand Tools." Vol 1 *Epidemiology.* Cincinnati, Ohio: 1982; DHHS (NIOSH) No 82-118.
8. Stewart, A. M. and Goda, D. F. "Vibration Syndrome." *Brit. J. Ind. Med.* 1970; 27:19–27.
9. Taylor, W. and Pelmear, P. L. eds. *Vibration White Finger in Industry.* London: Academic Press, 1975:166.
10. Kyriakides, K. *Survey of Exposure to Hand-Arm Vibration in Great Britain.* 1988. Health Safety Exec.
11. Bednall, A. W. "Hand-Arm Vibration in Great Britain." *J. Low. Freq. Noise Vib.* 1989; 8 (3): 81–86.
12. Seyring, M. "Maladies From Work With Compressed Air Drills." *Bull. Hyg.* 1931; 6:25.
13. Cummins, R. C. "Dead Hand": A Lesion Produced by Rapid Vibration. *Irish J. Med. Sci.* 1940; April: 171–175.
14. Gurdjian, E. S.; Walker, L. W. "Traumatic Vasospastic Disease of the Hand (White Fingers), With Particular Reference to Biopsy Findings." Jama 1945; 129:668–672.

15. Hunt, J. H. "Raynaud's Phenomenon in Workmen Using Vibrating Instruments." *Proc. Roy. Soc. Med.* 1936; 30:171-178.
16. McLaren, J. W. "Disability of Workers Using Pneumatic Drills, With Special Reference to Radiological Changes. *Lancet* 1937; 2:1296-1299.
17. Hunter, D.; McLaughlin, A. I. G.; Perry, K. M. A. "Clinical Effects of the Use of Pneumatic Tools." *Brit. J. Ind. Med.* 1945; 2:10-16.
18. Magos, L. and Okos, G. "Raynaud's Phenomenon. The Situation in the Hungarian Iron, Steel and Engineering Industry." *Arch. Environ. Health* 1963; 7:341-345.
19. Brocklehurst, T. "Pseudo-Raynaud's Disease due to Electric Vibratory Tools." *Med. Press* 1945; 213:10-11.
20. Biden-Steel, K., and King, F. H. " 'Dead Hand' in Operators Using Electrically Driven Cutting Tools." 1947; 218-144.
21. Agate, J. N., and Druett, H. A. "A Method for Studying Vibrations Transmitted to the Hands." *Brit. J. Ind. Med.* 1946; 3:159-166.
22. Agate, J. N.; Druett, H. A.; Tombleson, J. B. L. "Raynaud's Phenomenon in Grinders of Small Metal Castings." *Brit. J. Ind. Med.* 1946; 3:167-174.
23. Agate, J. N.; and Druett, H. A. "A Study of Portable Vibrating Tools in Relation to the Clinical Effects Which They Produce." *Brit. J. Ind. Med.* 1947; 4:141-163.
24. Agate, J. N. "An Outbreak of Cases of Raynaud's Phenomenon of Occupational Orgin." *Brit. J. Ind. Med.* 1949; 6:144-163.
25. Oliver, T. P.; Pethybridge, R. J.; Lumley, K. P. S. "Vibration White Finger in Dockyard Workers." *Arh. hig. rada. toksikol.* 1979; 30:683-693.
26. Bovenzi, M.; Petronio, L.; DiMarino, F. "Epidemiological Survey of Shipyard Workers Exposed to Hand-Arm Vibration." *Int. Arch. Occup. Environ. Health* 1980; 46:251-266.
27. Wasserman et al: "Vibration White Finger Disease in U.S. Workers."
28. Behrens, B.; Taylor, W.; Wilcox, T.; Miday, R.; Spaeth, S.; Burg, J. "Vibration Syndrome in Chipping and Grinding Workers." III. *Epidemiology. J. Med.* 1984; 26(10): 769-773.
29. Jepson R. P. "Raynaud's Phenomenon in Workers With Vibratory Tools." *Brit. J. Ind. Med.* 1954; 11:180-185.
30. Williams, N. and Riegert, A. L. "Raynaud's Phenomenon of Occupational Origin in Uranium Miners." In: *Proceedings of the 13th International Congress on Occupational Health*. New York, 1962:819-825.
31. Ashe, W. F.; Cook, W. T.; Old, J. W. "Raynaud's Phenomenon of Occupational Origin." *Arch, Environ. Health.* 1962; 5:333-343.
32. Ashe, W. F., and Williams, N. "Occupational Raynaud's." *Arch. Environ. Health* 1964; 9:425-433.
33. Lindstrom, I. M. "Vibration Injury in Rock Drillers, Chisellers and Grinders." In: Wasserman, D. E.; Taylor, W.; Curry, M. G., eds., *Proceedings of the International Occupational Hand-Arm Conference*. Cincinatti, Ohio: 1977; 77-84. DHHS (NIOSH) publication No. 77-170.
34. Chatterjee, D. S.; Petrie, A.; Taylor, W. "Prevalence of Vibration Induced White Finger in Fluorspar Mines in Weardale." *Brit J. Ind. Med.* 1978; 35:208-218.
35. Rodgers, L. A.; Eglin, D.; Hart, W. F. D. "Rock-Drill Vibration and White Fingers in Miners." In: Brammer, A. J., and Taylor, W., eds. *Vibration Effects on the Hand and Arm in Industry*. New York: Wiley, 1982:317-323.

36. Iwata, H. "Effects of Rock Drills on Operators. Part 2. Survey and Examination on Raynaud's Phenomenon." *Ind. Health* 1968; 6:37-47.
37. Matsumoto, T.; Yamada, S.; Hisanga, N. "On Vibration Hazards in Rock-Drill Operators of a Metal Mine." *Jap. J. Ind. Health* 1977; 19:256-265.
38. Moon, Y. H.; Roh, J. H.; Cheon, Y. H. "Vibration Hazards in Rock-Drill Operators of the Anthracine Mine." In: Proceedings of the 10th Asian Conference on Occupational Health 1982; 1:402-407.
39. Hutton, S. G.; and Brubaker, R. L. "Vibration Effects on Mine Workers." *CIM Bulletin* 1982; 75 (838): 85-93.
40. Brubaker, R. L.; Mackenzie, C. J. G.; Hutton, S. G. "A study of Vibration White Finger Disease Rock Drillers." *J. Low. Freq. Noise Vib.* 1985; 4 (2): 52-65.
41. Pelmear, P. L., Taraschuk, I.; Leong, D.; Wong, L. "Cold Water Immersion Test in Hand-Arm Vibration Exposure." *J. Low Freq. Noise Vib.* 1985; 4:89-97.
42. Pelmear, P. L.; Leong, D.; Taraschuk, I.; Wong, L. "Hand-Arm Vibration Syndrome in Foundrymen and Hard Rock Miners." *J. Low Freq. Noise Vib.* 1986; 5 (1): 26-43.
43. Brubaker, R. L.; Mackenzie, C. J. G.; Hutton, S. G. "Vibration-Induced White Finger Among Selected Underground Rock Drillers in British Columbia." *Scand. J. Work. Environ. Health* 1986; 12:296-300.
44. Pelmear, P. L.; Roos, J.; Leong, D.; Wong, L. "Cold Provocation Test Results From a 1985 Survey of Hard-Rock Miners in Ontario." *Scand. J. Work. Environ. Health* 1987; 13:343-347.
45. Wasserman, D. E.; Behrens, V. J.; Pelmear, P. L.; et al.: "Hand-Arm Vibration Syndrome in a Group of U.S. Uranium Miners Exposed to Hand-Arm Vibration." *Appl. Occup. Environ. Hyg.* 1991; 6 (3): 183-187.
46. Taylor, W.; Wasserman, D.; Behrens, V.; Reynolds, D.; Samueloff, S. "Effect of the Air Hammer on the Hands of Stonecutters. The Limestone Quarries of Bedford, Indiana, Revisited." *Brit. J. Ind. Med.* 1984; 41:289-295.
47. Bovenzi, M.; Franzinelli, A.; Strambi, F. "Prevalence of Vibration-Induced White Finger and Assessments of Vibration Exposure Among Travertine Workers in Italy." *Int. Arch. Occup. Environ. Health* 1988; 61:25-34.
48. Musson, Y.; Burdorf, A.; Van Drimmelen, D. "Exposure to Shock and Vibration and Symptoms in Workers Using Impact Power Tools." *Ann. Occup. Hyg.* 1989; 33 (1):85-96.
49. Walker, D. D.; Jones, B.; Ogston, S.; Tasker, E. G.; Robinson, A. J. "A Study of White Finger in the Gas Industry." *Brit. J. Ind. Med.* 1985; 42: 672-677.
50. Nilsson, T.; Burström, L.; Hagberg, M. "Risk Assessment of Vibration Exposure and White Fingers Among Platers." *Int. Arch. Occup. Environ. Health* 1989; 61:473-481
51. Pelmear, P. L.; Taylor, W.; Pearson, J. C. G. "Raynaud's Phenomenon in Grinders." In: Taylor, W., and Pelmear, P. L., eds. *Vibration White Finger in Industry.* London: Academic Press, 1975; 21-30.
52. Starck, J. Färkkilä, M.; Aatola, S., Pyykkö, I., Korhonen, O. "Vibration Syndrome and Vibration in Pedestal Grinding." *Brit J. Ind. Med.* 1983; 40:426-433.
53. Grounds, M. D. "Raynaud's Phenomenon in Users of Chain Saws." *Med. J. Aust.* 1964; 1:270-272.

54. Miura, T.; Kimura, K.; Tominaga, Y.; Kimotsuki, K. "On the Raynaud's Phenomenon of Occupational Origin due to Vibrating Tools—Its Incidence in Japan." *Report of the Institute for Science and Labour*, Tokyo, Japan. No. 65:1-11.
55. Axelsson, S. A. "Analysis of Vibration in Power Saws." No. 59, Skogshogskolan, Royal College of Forestry Monograph, Stockholm. 1968.
56. Kylin, B.; Gerhardsson, G.; Hansson, J.; et al. "Halso—Och Miljoundersokning Bland Skogsorb Etare Al—Rapports." 1968.
57. Barnes, R.; Longley, E. O.; Smith, A. R. B.; Allen, J. G. "Vibration Disease." *Med. J. Aust.* 1969; 1:901-905.
58. Taylor, W.; Pearson, J.; Kell, R. L.; Keighley, G. D. "Vibration Syndrome in Forestry Commission Chain Saw Operators." *Brit. J. Ind. Med.* 1971; 28:83-89.
59. Taylor, W.; Pelmear, P. L.; Pearson, J. "Raynaud's Phenomenon in Forestry Chain Saw Operators." In: Taylor, W.; ed. *The Vibration Syndrome*, London: Academic Press, 1974:121-139.
60. Hellstrom, B.; and Andersen, K. L. "Vibration Injuries in Norwegian Forest Workers." *Brit. J. Ind. Med.* 1972; 29:255-263.
61. Taylor, W.; Pelmear, P. L.; Pearson, J. C. G. "A Longitudinal Study of Raynaud's Phenomenon in Chain Saw Operators." In: Taylor, W., and Pelmear, P. L.,eds. *Vibration White Finger in Industry*. London: Academic Press, 1975:15-20.
62. Theriault, G.; DeGuire, L.; Gingras, S.; Larouche, G. "Raynaud's Phenomenon in Forest Workers in Quebec." *CMAJ* 1982; 126(12): 1404-1408.
63. Pyykkö, I. "The Prevalence and Symptoms of Traumatic Vasospastic Disease Among Lumberjacks in Finland. A Field Study." *Work Environ. Health* 1974; 11:118-131.
64. Futatsuka, M. and Ueno, T,. "Vibration Exposure and Vibration-Induced White Finger due to Chain Saw Operation." *J. Occup. Med.* 1985; 27(4): 257-264.
65. Futatsuka, M., and Ueno, T. "A Follow-up Study of Vibration-Induced White Finger due to Chain-Saw Operation." *Scand. J. Work Environ. Health.* 1986; 12:304-306.
66. Futatsuka, M.; Ueno, T.; Sakurai, T. "Cohort Study of Vibration-Induced White Finger Among Japanese Forest Workers Over 30 Years." *Ind. Arch. Environ. Health* 1989; 61:503-506.
67. Pyykkö I.; Korhonen, O. S.; Färkkilä, M. A.; Starck, J. P.; Aatola, S. A. "A Longitudinal Study of the Vibration Syndrome in Finnish Forestry Workers." In: Brammer, A. J., and Taylor, W., eds. *Vibration Effects of the Hand and Arm in Industry*. New York: John Wiley & Sons, 1982:157-167.
68. Pyykkö, I,; Korhonen, O.; Färkkilä, M.; Starck, J.; Aatola, S.; Jäntti, V. "Vibration Syndrome Among Finnish Forest Workers, a Follow-up From 1972 to 1983." *Scand. J. Work Environ. Health* 1986; 12:307-312.
69. Brubaker, R. L.; Mackenzie. C. J. G.; Eng. P. R.; Bates. V. V.; "Vibration White Finger Disease Among Tree Fellers in British Columbia." *J. Occup. Med.* 1983; 25(5):403-408.
70. Brubaker. R. L.; Mackenzie. C. J. G.; Hertzman. C.; Hutton. S. G.; Slakov. J. "Longitudinal Study of Vibration-Induced White Finger Among Coastal Fallers in British Columbia. *Scand. J. Work. Environ. Health* 1987; 13:505-308.
71. Pelnar, P. V.; Gibbs, G. W.; Pathak, B. P. "A Pilot Investigation of the Vibration Syndrome in Forestry Workers of Eastern Canada." In: Brammer, A. J.; and Taylor, W,

eds. *Vibration Effects on the Hand and Arm in Industry.* New York: John Wiley & Sons, 1982:173-187.

72. Miyashika, K.; Shiomi, S.; Itoh, N.; Vasamaku, T.; Iwata, H. "Epidemiological Study of Vibration Syndrome in Response to Total Hand-Tool Operating Time." *Brit. J. Ind. Med.* 1983; 40:92-98.

73. Futatsuka, M.; Yasutake, N.; Sakurai, T.; Matsumoto, T. "Comparative Study of Vibration Disease Among Operators of Vibrating Tools by Factor Analysis." *Brit. J. Ind. Med.* 1985; 42:260-266.

74. Bentley, S.; O'Conner, D. E.; Lord, P; Edmonds, O. P.; "Vibration White Finger in Motorcycle Speedway Riders." In: Brammer, A. J.; and Taylor, W., eds. *Vibration Effects on the Hand and Arm in Industry.* New York: John Wiley & Sons, 1982:189-192.

75. Futatsuka, M. "A Study on the Vibration Hazards due to Using Brush Cutters." *Jpn. J. Health* 1979; 21:269-273.

76. Futatsuka, M. "Epidemiological Studies of Vibration Disease due to Brush Saw Operation." *Ind. Arch. Occup. Environ. Health* 1984; 54:251-260.

77. Hisashige, A.; Kume, I.; Ogawa, T.; Taniguchi, K.; Nakagivi, S.; Aoyama, H. "A Study on Vibration Syndrome Among Brush Cleaner Operators." *Jpn. J. Ind. Health* 1979; 21:683-684.

78. Itoh, N.; Kasamatsu, T.; Shiomi, S.; Iwata, H. "Vibration Disease due to Grass Cutters." *Jpn. J. Ind. Health* 1978; 29:451-452.

79. Fatatsuka, "Epidemiological Studies."

80. Bovenzi, M.; Peretti, A.; Zadini, A.; Betta, A.; Passeri, A. C. "Physiological Reactions During Brush Saws Operation." *Ind. Arch. Occup. Environ. Health* 1990; 62:445-449.

81. Taylor, W.; Pelmear, P. L.; Pearson, J. C. G. "Vibration-Induced White Finger Epidemiology." In: Taylor, W.; and Pelmear, P.L.; eds. *Vibration White Finger in Industry.* London: Academic Press, 1975; 1-13.

82. Stewart, A. M. and Goda, D. F. "Vibration Syndrome." *Brit. J. Ind. Med.* 1970:27; 19-27.

83. Riddle, H. F. V. and Taylor, W. "Vibration-Induced White Finger Among Chain Sawyers Nine Years After the Introduction of Anti-Vibration Measures." In: Brammer, A. J. and Taylor, W, eds. *Vibration Effects on the Hand and Arm in Industry.* New York: John Wiley & Sons 1982:169-172.

84. Hursh. H. J. "Vibration-Induced White Finger—Reversible or Not. A Preliminary Report." In: Brammer. A. J.; and Taylor, W.; eds. *Vibration effects on the Hand and Arm in Industry.* New York: John Wiley & Sons, 1982:156-167.

85. Pyykkö, I.; Korhonen, O. S.; Färkkilä, M. A.; Starck, J. P.; Aatola, S. A. "A Longitudinal Study of the Vibration Syndrome in Finnish Forestry Workers." In: Brammer, A. J.; and Taylor, W.; eds. *Vibration Effects on the Hand and Arm in Industry.* New York: John Wiley & Sons, 1982:156-167.

86. Futatsuka, M.; Ueno, T.; Sakurai, T. "Follow-up Study of Vibration Induce White Finger in Chain Saw Operators." *Brit. J. Ind. med.* 1985; 42:267-271.

87. Ekenvall, L. and Carlsson, A. "Vibration White Finger: A Follow-up Study" *Brit. J. Ind. Med.* 1987; 44:476-478.

88. Olsen, N. and Nielsen, S. L. "Vasoconstrictor Response to Cold in Forestry Workers; A Prospective Study." *Brit. J. Ind. Med.* 1988; 45:39-42.

89. James, P. B.; and Galloway, R. W. "Brachial Arteriography in Vibration Induced White Finger." In: Taylor, W.; and Pelmear, P. L., eds. *Vibration White Finger in Industry.* London: Academic Press, 1975:31–42.

90. Wasserman, D. E.; and Taylor, W. "Historical Perspectives in Occupational Medicine: Lessons From Hand-Arm Vibration Syndrome Research." *Amer. J. Ind. Med.* 1991; 19:539–546.

91. Dandanell, R. and Engstrom, K. "Vibration From Riveting Tools in the Frequency Range 6 Hz–10 MHz and Raynaud's Phenomenon." *Scand. J. Work. Environ. Health.* 1986; 12:338–342.

92. Lundström, R. and Lindmark, A. "Effects of Local Vibration on Tactile Perception in the Hands of Dentists. *J. Low. Freq. Noise Vib.* 1982; 1:1–11.

93. Starck, J. "Characteristics of Vibration, Hand Grip Force, and Hearing Loss in Vibration Syndrome." Helsinki, Finland; University of Kisupio; 1984. Dissertation.

94. Pelmear, P. L.; Taylor, W.; Nagalingam, M.; Fung, D. "Measurement of Vibration of Hand-Held Tools: Weighted or Unweighted? *J. Occup. Med.* 1989; 31(11):902–908.

95. "Criteria for a Recommended Standard. Occupational Exposure to Hand-Arm Vibration." 1989 DHHS (NIOSH) publication 89-106.

8

Hand-Arm Vibration and Work-Related Disorders of the Upper Limb

R. G. Radwin, T. J. Armstrong, E. VanBergeijk

This chapter discusses causes and prevention of acute and chronic upper limb disorders associated with manual work and hand-transmitted vibration. Ergonomic stresses include posture, repetitive motion, forceful exertions, contact stresses, and cold temperatures, in addition to vibration. These stresses are recognized as risk factors for upper extremity cumulative trauma disorders (CTDs). Cumulative trauma disorders include disorders of the tendons, nerves, bones, and muscles that are caused, aggravated, and precipitated from repeated exposure to these stresses. Hand-tool operators are often confronted with a number of these ergonomic and physical stresses, including hand-arm vibration (HAV). Although ergonomic stresses are recognized risk factors, there are insufficient data to predict the effects of changing any one of them on the risk of incurring a CTD. The ability to predict is further complicated by the occurrence of more than one factor in a given work situation.

The relative effects of hand-transmitted vibration and other ergonomic stress factors are often difficult to separate because many jobs using vibrating hand tools also involve considerable use of the upper limb. For instance, vibrating hand-tool operators may also have to assume awkward postures dictated by a specific tool-handle location and work piece orientation. Vibrating power-tool handles and triggers may introduce contact stress from sharp edges against the fingers or palm. The hands may also be exposed to cold air produced from pneumatic tool exhaust outlets.

Furthermore, ergonomic stress factors can adversely affect vibration transmission and exposure. For example, forceful exertions will result in increased vibration transfer to the tool operator's hand and arm because of improved coupling between the vibrating handle and the hand. Highly repetitive work can affect vibration exposure through accumulated doses of repeated vibration exposures. These inter-

122

actions have certainly complicated the study of ergonomic stress factors and their combined effects with hand-transmitted vibration.

RELATIONSHIP BETWEEN UPPER EXTREMITY CTDs AND HAV

Until recently, scientific attention has focused primarily on vascular vibration disorders such as vibration white finger (VWF),[1-3] bone and joint deformations,[4] autonomic disturbances,[5] perception,[6, 7] discomfort,[8] and other miscellaneous abnormalities.[9] Musculoskeletal and peripheral nerve disorders associated with HAV, however, are now beginning to gain recognition.

Carpal tunnel syndrome (CTS), a neuropathy of the median nerve at the wrist, is a commonly cited CTD associated with operating vibrating hand tools.[10, 11] Carpal tunnel syndrome is characterized by tingling, numbness, and pain in the areas of the hand innervated by the median nerve. Separating neurological disorders, such as CTS, from vascular disorders, such as VWF, has been difficult since a number of the early symptoms for both disorders are similar. Hence the effects of CTS and hand-arm vibration syndrome (HAVS) are often confounded.[12] Epidemiological studies of degenerative changes in the hand-arm system caused by vibration[13, 14] have proved it difficult to differentiate between the direct effects of vibration and those of heavy manual work involving forceful and repetitive movements.

Seppalainen[15] compared the results of neurological examinations of nine lumberjacks who used chain saws regularly, and eight workers who regularly worked with pneumatic rock drills. Seven of the drill users complained of paresthesia and other neurological deficits. Although no formal description of the lumberjack and rock driller jobs were provided, it can be assumed that in addition to vibration, these workers also performed repeated and sustained exertions and possibly exerted high forces.

Rothfleisch and Sherman[16] studied the factors associated with CTS for 25 hands in 16 workers at an automobile assembly plant. Each of these workers at some time used pneumatic tools, which were reported vibrating between 8 Hz and 33 Hz. They also found that awkward positioning of the hand and wrist while performing their tasks was a common factor. This study again showed that ergonomic and vibration factors occur together, and that their effects were not easily separated.

Cannon et al.[17] performed a retrospective case controlled study on 30 workers with CTS. The most significant factor was the use of vibrating hand tools (odds ratio 7.0). Although performing repetitive motion tasks was less important (odds ratio 2.1), it can be assumed that exposure to vibration also involved intensive use of the hands. Therefore, sustained exertions, high forces, and posture may account for some or most of the apparent vibration effect.

A cross-sectional study of 652 active workers in 39 jobs in seven different U.S. industrial plants was performed in order to investigate occupational risk factors of

CTS.[18, 19] Four of the jobs that were classified as high-force involved nearly continuous exposure to vibration (buffing, grinding, cutting) while none of the control jobs involved vibration exposure. The crude odds ratio for the jobs classified high-force, high-repetitive with vibration versus the control jobs was 11.3. The odds ratio for the high-force, high-repetitive jobs with no vibration versus the same control jobs was only 5.9. When high-force, high-repetitive jobs with vibration were compared with those without vibration, the odds ratio was 1.9. These data suggest that the risk of CTS for low-repetitive, low-force work is increased by a factor of 6 and that the risk of CTS for high-force, high-repetitive work is elevated by a factor of 2 when accompanied with nearly continuous vibration exposure. While hand and wrist tendinitis were highly associated with high-force, high-repetitive work with an odds ratio of 18.9 ($p < .01$), no association with vibration was found.

ERGONOMIC STRESS FACTORS ASSOCIATED WITH POWER HAND TOOLS

If physical exertions are sufficiently frequent, long, and forceful, or they occur in certain postures, they are performed in cold environments, or they result in sufficient contact stress, a worker can develop pain and impairment in the upper limb. These disorders have specific names, depending on the location and the tissues involved, but it suffices to simply refer to them collectively as CTDs. The risk of incurring a CTD may be altered by congenital factors, chronic diseases, acute injuries, and physiological states. This discussion will focus on the work-related factors: 1) repetitiveness, 2) forcefulness, 3) posture, 4) contact stress, and 5) cold temperature.

Repetitiveness

Repetitiveness refers to the number of exertions repeated per unit time, and how long exertions are maintained. The relationship between the degree of repetitiveness and the risk of a CTD is not yet known. As early as 1927, Obolenskaja and Goljanitzki[20] suggested that high rates of work, 7,600 to 12,000 exertions per shift, was a major factor in 189 cases of tenosynovitis of the upper extremities among a group of 700 packers in a tea factory. Hammer[21] suggested that human tendons do not tolerate more than 1,500 to 2,000 exertions per hour. Tichauer[22] concluded 5,000 exertions per day was sufficient to produce injury of the median nerve.

In many instances, it can be shown that the number of exertions is related to the number of parts produced per unit time, or the number of work cycles. Luopajarvi et al.,[23] concluded that the prevalence of muscle-tendon syndromes in the hands of assembly-line packers were related to operators keeping up with machine paces of 25,000 cycles per day. Kuorinka and Koskinen[24] found the symptoms of muscle-tendon disorders increased as the number of parts handled per year increased from less than 200,000 to more than 300,000. Silverstein et al.[25] found increases in the risk of CTS and tendinitis with fundamental work cycles of less than 30 seconds that were performed for more than 50 percent of the time.

Forcefulness

Forcefulness is the amount of force exerted using the hands for lifting, moving or holding something. Many investigators only talk about forceful exertions without actually measuring them.[26-30] Some investigators use surface electromyography and job analysis to estimate hand forces in work. Armstrong and Chaffin[31] found that persons with CTS tend to exert 18 percent more force than age, gender, and job-matched controls. Silverstein et al.[32] estimated forces using surface electromyography, but grouped their study population into two groups with high and low-force exposure. They found that the risk of tendinitis and CTS increased 29 and 15 times, respectively, with high force and repetitiveness. Recently small, flat sensors that attach to the hands have been demonstrated as being useful for measuring finger forces produced during carrying and gripping activities.[33] It is anticipated that these sensors will be used in future ergonomics investigations for assessing hand force.

Posture

Posture is the position assumed by the body, or specific body parts, during a task. Flexion and extreme extension of the wrist compresses and stretches the median nerve, tendons, and tendon sheaths, and is associated with CTS.[34-43] Ulnar deviation of the wrist stretches the abductor and extensor tendons of the thumb and is associated with de Quervain's disease.[44-53] Extreme forearm rotation stretches the tendonous attachments of the forearm flexor and extensor muscles and is associated with epicondylitis.[54-56] Extreme elbow flexion stretches the median nerve and is associated with cubital tunnel syndrome.[57-62] These postures are illustrated in Figure 8-1

Contact Stress

Contact stress is produced when the body comes into contact with an external object. Contact stress is related to the force and area of contact. The smaller the contact area, the greater the stress concentration for a given force level. Contact with the lateral sides of the fingers is associated with digital neuritis[63,64] and contact with the palmar sides of the fingers is associated with trigger finger[65,66] while contact with the base of the palm is associated with CTS.[67-71]

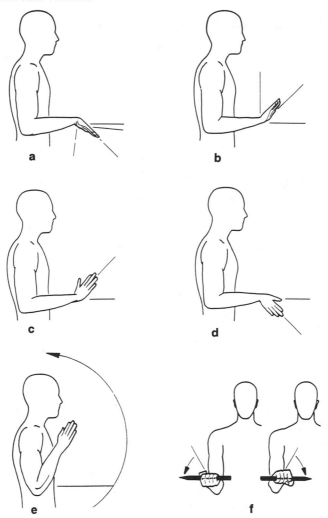

FIGURE 8-1. Stressful elbow and wrist postures include flexion (a) and extreme extension of the wrist (b), radial deviation of the wrist (c), ulnar deviation of the wrist (d), extreme flexion of the elbow (e), and extreme forearm rotation (f).

Cold Temperature

Cold temperature affects sensitivity and manipulative ability of the hands.[72-77] Lowered skin temperatures can increase forcefulness and accentuate possible neurological symptoms due to CTDs. In addition, there is evidence that extreme cooling may directly produce tendinitis.[78]

ERGONOMIC STRESS FACTORS
AND THEIR EFFECTS ON VIBRATION
TRANSMISSION AND EXPOSURE

The previous section described recognized ergonomics stress factors associated with hand-tool operation. Often these stress factors are accompanied by vibration. Power hand tools impart vibration to the hand and arm by way of (1) the worker-tool interface, (2) the intrinsic tool properties, and (3) the tool–material interface.

Worker–Tool Interface

The worker-tool interface is the path vibration energy takes between the source and the human operator. It describes the interaction between the hand tool and the operator. The worker-tool interface may involve the use of handles (or lack of using them) or other parts of the tool in contact with the hands and body. Handle location and the type of tool can have a dramatic effect on the level of vibration transmitted to the operator. Vibration measurements made from a large chipping hammer[79] in the y-axis over a frequency range of 6.3 Hz–1,000 Hz, taken at points where workers normally grip these tools running at full throttle, indicated that the acceleration ratio between the chisel end to rear handle was approximately 78:1 (23,400 m/s^2 at the chisel and 299 m/s^2 at the rear handle). These actual measurements are probably on the high side compared to more recent studies. The same study found that rear-handle acceleration levels for a small stone chipper were 2:1 (4,840 m/s^2 at the chisel and 2,010 m/s^2 at the rear handle), apparently due to very little mass damping for this lightweight tool.

Work standards and individual work methods are another aspect of the worker-tool interface. One study found the prevalence of HAVS was greater among incentive workers than among hourly workers.[80] The characteristics of incentive work were associated with shortened latencies and increased severity. The report suggested that the intensity of incentive work resulted in increased vibration transmission and therefore exposure, presumably due to increased grip exertions and the resulting improved coupling between the hand and the power tool.

Daily vibration exposure is directly related to the repetitive nature of the work or the number of operations per day. The results of the following study by Radwin and Armstrong[81] illustrate how vibration exposure is related to repetitive work involving installation of screws on an electrical appliance assembly line. This study was undertaken to investigate the contribution of pneumatic screwdrivers to CTDs, which were a major cause of lost time and workers' compensation at the facility. High vibration-exposure levels were considered to be due to the highly repetitive nature of this work.

Figure 8-2 illustrates a typical work station on the assembly line. Workers operated the in-line tools on a horizontal surface at elbow height while seated at a

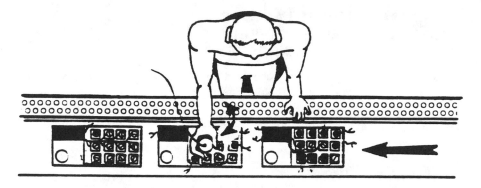

FIGURE 8-2.   Representative bench assembly work station. Workers seated alongside of the
conveyor load pneumatic screwdrivers with screws scattered along a perforated tray in front of the
conveyor. The loaded screwdriver is repeatedly moved between the tray to a threaded hole where a
screw is installed. Reproduced with permission from Radwin, R. G. and Armstrong, T. J.,
"Assessment of Hand Vibration Exposure on an Assembly Line," *American Industrial Hygiene
Association Journal*: Vol.46(4): 211-219 (1985).

work bench. Hand and wrist posture was not considered a problem here since
workers generally did not have to flex, hyperextend, deviate their wrists, rotate
their forearms, or elevate their elbows. Employees were paid on a group incentive,
and operators often backed up co-workers when they fell behind to maintain the
line production rate. The average production rate was 2.9 units per minute for these
highly repetitive tasks.

Vibration exposure was measured using observation samples of tool vibration
obtained on the assembly line from individual work stations and predicting daily
exposure from these samples for each position on the assembly line. The screwdrivers were push-to-start, torque-controlled tools designed to start when the bit or
socket was depressed and stop when this pressure was removed. A ratcheting clutch
mechanism caused the motor to slip when a screw was tightened to the set torque.
This torque was in the 0.9 Nm (80 in lbs) range. Ratcheting clutches produce
vibration only after the tool has tightened a fastener. Figure 8-3 illustrates a typical
ratcheting clutch pneumatic power-tool mechanism.

Vibration recordings obtained by attaching an accelerometer to the screwdrivers
indicated that there were two distinct phases associated with the screwdriver
operation. Figure 8-4 is a representative acceleration record. The first portion of
the wave form was produced during the "run phase," corresponding to when the
screwdriver was free running during screw pick-up and when driving a screw. The
second portion, or "clutch phase," corresponded to the screwdriver clutch mechanism slippage when the screw was tightened to the set torque. Visual inspection of
the wave form in Figure 8-4 clearly reveals that the vibration produced during the

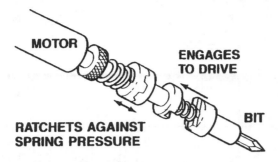

FIGURE 8-3. Details of a power tool using a ratcheting clutch shut-off mechanism. Ratcheting mechanism causes the tool to vibrate when the drive becomes disengaged at the set torque level.

"clutch phase" was much greater in amplitude and fundamentally lower in frequency than during the "run phase." Spectral analysis confirmed that the run phase contained vibration widely distributed between 31.5 Hz and 1,000 Hz for a peak acceleration amplitude of 10 m/s^2, while the clutch phase consisted of vibration predominantly at 100 Hz for a peak acceleration amplitude more than 100 m/s^2.

Plotting predicted total daily exposure versus the number of screws per cycle, as a measure of repetitiveness, reveals a direct relationship between repetitiveness and vibration exposure (see Figure 8-5). Hence workers exposed to greater repetitive stresses were also subject to greater exposures of vibration. Since this study was conducted, most of the screwdriving tasks at that plant have been eliminated due to changes in product technology that have eliminated most of the screws from the circuits. This has nearly eliminated vibration exposure.

Modifications in work methods can affect vibration-exposure levels produced as well as vibration-exposure patterns. Vibration exposure may also be controlled through work-method modifications such as redesigning production processes for reducing or eliminating vibrating hand tools, redistributing the work among workers, and use of external tool support devices for reducing grip force or eliminating the need to hold tools when in use. Vibration exposure can also be lowered using worker rotation and work enlargement methods for controlling highly repetitive motions.

In addition to the obvious effects on metabolic demand, forcefulness also increases vibration transmission to the hand. Pyykkö et al.[82] attached accelerometers to the skin at a number of locations along the hand and arm. Using an electromagnetic shaker vibrating at swept frequencies, they found the hand-arm system behaved as a low-pass filter where vibration transmission measured at the wrist was less attenuated than at the upper arm and elbow for frequencies above 100 Hz. Increased grip compression force improved transmission to the upper extremity. Iwata et al.[83] and Reynolds[84] showed similar results.

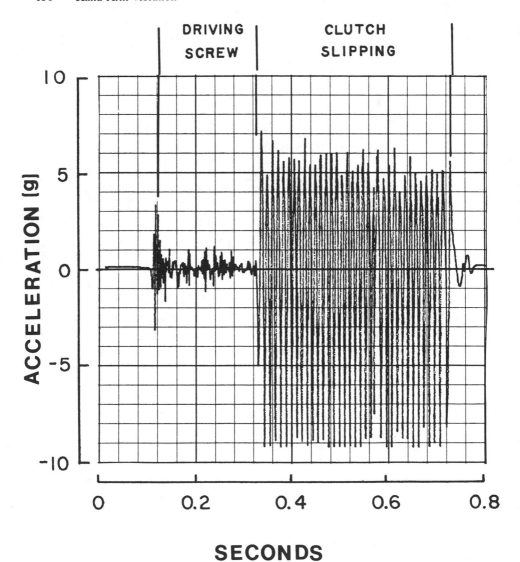

FIGURE 8-4.   Representative clutch shut-off pneumatic screwdriver acceleration wave form. Reproduced with permission from Radwin, R. G. and Armstrong, T. J., "Assessment of Hand Vibration Exposure on an Assembly Line." *American Industrial Hygiene Association Journal*: Vol.46(4): 211–219 (1985).

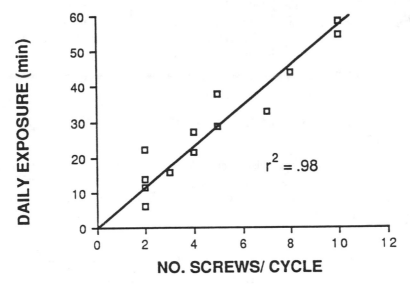

FIGURE 8-5. Plot of predicted total daily vibration exposure versus repetitiveness, indicated by the number of screws installed per cycle for each work station.

Intrinsic Tool Properties

Vibration is an outcome of power hand-tool operation and may be the actual desired action of a particular tool or a by-product of its operation. The vibration level produced depends on intrinsic tool properties, including size, weight, method of propulsion, and the tool drive mechanism. Continuous vibration is inherent in reciprocating and rotary power tools. Impulsive vibration is produced by tools operating by shock and impact action, such as impact wrenches or chippers. The tool power source, such as air power, electricity, or hydraulics, can also affect vibration.

Accessory attachments may become a source of vibration if they fit improperly or cause a tool to become unbalanced. An example is a loosely fitting extension shaft on a nut runner, causing a tool usually not considered a vibrating hand tool to produce considerable vibration from the wobbling action of the rotating spindle. Tools requiring maintenance, or tools that become unbalanced, are also potential sources of vibration. Some tools are specifically designed to minimize vibration.

Tool–Material Interface

Vibration is generated at the tool–material interface by cutting, grinding, drilling, or other actions. Vibration levels are affected by work piece material properties, disk abrasives, abrasive surface area, and fastener type. Material properties include hardness or surface characteristics such as roughness, or shape. Reducing a sanding pad grit abrasiveness may decrease the overall vibration level; however, it is important to be sure this doesn't affect the force requirements or increase vibration-exposure time and repetitiveness by increasing the amount of sanding necessary for accomplishing the task.

VIBRATION EFFECTS ON CTD STRESS FACTORS

There are two possible mechanisms for HAV and CTS. Peripheral nerve damage may result from a primary lesion caused directly by vibration, or indirectly through secondary disturbances caused from damage of the circulatory or musculoskeletal systems. There is evidence, however, that vascular and neurological disorders associated with HAV may develop independently.[85] In the assessment of neurological disorders by electrophysiological studies Lukás[86] drew attention to the three regions that are a possible source of secondary neurogenic lesions: (1) the cervical and upper thoracic regions, (2) the elbow joint, and (3) the carpal tunnel and ulnar nerve region. It was not possible to prove that exposure to vibration was the primary cause of the observed electromyogram (EMG) changes.

Studies conducted by Radwin et al.[87, 88] of the short-term neuromuscular effects of hand-tool vibration have demonstrated that hand-tool vibration can introduce disturbances in neuromuscular force control resulting in excessive grip exertions when holding a vibrating handle. Since forceful exertions are a commonly cited factor of chronic muscle, tendon, and nerve disorders of the upper extremities, vibrating hand-tool operation may increase the risk of CTDs through increased grip force. Furthermore these studies provide evidence that upper extremity CTDs involving peripheral nerves, such as CTS, may occur indirectly through increased forcefulness, as an alternative to direct injury to the nerve tissue arising from the vibratory energy.

Neuromuscular effects of vibration were recognized as early as 1860 when Rood[89] observed while grinding a glass microscope slide that it vibrated and he experienced "...a numbness, and, at times, an absolute inability to relax the grasp." Rood went on to state, "it seems as though an involuntary contraction of the muscles had been affected by the vibratory action."

Vibration can introduce disturbances in muscular control by way of a reflex mediated through the response of muscle spindles to the vibration stimulus. Using decerebrate cat preparations, Matthews[90] attached a vibrator to the fully innervated soleus muscle tendon and reported a reflexive response that increased tension in the vibrated muscle by increasing vibration amplitude and increasing frequency between 50 Hz and 300 Hz. This reflex, known as the tonic vibration reflex (TVR), has been observed in humans causing a gradual increase in activity of moderately active muscle having their tendons vibrated.[91, 92] The result is either slow joint motion or a corresponding change in active tension. The TVR offers an explanation for increased grip force when holding a vibrating handle.

In order to study the neuromuscular effects of vibration, a simulator was developed for laboratory experiments, capable of controlling load weight, posture, vibration frequency, magnitude, and direction, at typical hand-tool levels[93]. Typical vibrating hand tools used in manufacturing and assembly operations include small grinders, sanders, polishers, and impact wrenches. These tools typically weigh between 1.5 kg to 3.0 kg. Most tools have a rotary action producing a distinct dominant fundamental frequency at which acceleration is typically at least three-times (10 dB) greater than at other frequencies, indicating that sinusoidal wave forms adequately describe the vibration. Figure 8-6 shows dominant vibration frequencies and amplitudes for a number of representative tools often used in manufacturing. Dominant frequencies typically range between 20 Hz and 160 Hz.

Fourteen subjects operated the simulated hand tool, vibrating at 9.8 m/s² and 49 m/s² RMS (root mean square) acceleration magnitudes, 40 Hz and 160 Hz frequencies, in three orthogonal directions corresponding to the Internation Organization for Standardization (ISO) basicentric hand-arm coordinate system (ISO, 1984), and with 15 N and 30 N loads. The results of that study demonstrated that grip exertions increased with tool vibration. Average grip force increased from 25.3 N without vibration, to 32.1 N (27 percent) for vibration at 40 Hz, but only to 27.1 N (7 percent) for 160 Hz vibration. Average grip force also increased from 27.4 N for vibration amplitudes of 9.8 m/s² to 31.8 N for 49 m/s² amplitudes. Figure 8-7 is a

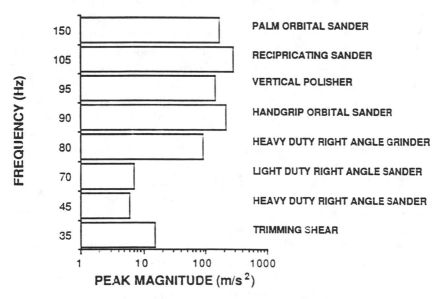

FIGURE 8-6.   Dominant vibration frequency characteristics for selected tools used in automobile manufacturing.

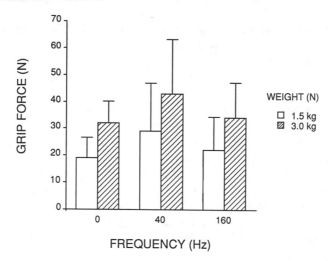

FIGURE 8-7.   Average grip force for 14 subjects holding a handle
weighing 1.5 kg or 3.0 kg and vibrating at 5 g RMS.

plot of grip force exerted by 14 subjects, averaged over vibration magnitude and
direction. The greatest average grip force increase observed was from 25.3 N
without vibration to 35.8 N (42 percent) for 40 Hz and 49 m/s² vibration. The
magnitude of this increase in grip force was similar to grip force for a twofold
increase in load weight where the average grip force increased from 22.5 N to 35.0
N (56 percent).

Another experiment was performed measuring hand flexor and extensor muscle
surface, EMGs, where subjects held a handle vibrating at 8 m/s² ISO weighted
acceleration,[94] for frequencies of 20 Hz, 40 Hz, 80 Hz, and 160 Hz, and grip forces
of 5 percent, 10 percent, and 15 percent of maximum voluntary contraction. The
results indicated that muscle responses were greatest at frequencies where grip
force was affected. Extensor activity was greater when the handle was vibrating
than without vibration. The effects were largest at 40 Hz vibration and 15 percent
maximum voluntary contraction in the vertical and longitudinal directions with
respect to the long axis of the forearm. These results advanced the argument that
the TVR was the cause of increased muscle contraction.

Westling and Johansson[95] showed that static force exerted when holding objects
between the thumb and forefinger was proportional to object weight and friction.
Local anesthesia of the index finger and thumb (5 mg Marcain/digit) resulted in
loss of sensitivity to object surface characteristics, and the tendency for exerting
nearly twice the unanesthetized force for a given object weight. As Rood[96] in 1860
also noted, vibration can cause numbness and diminish hand tactility. Vibration has
been shown to produce short-term sensory impairments.[97, 98] Recovery is exponen-
tial and can require more than 20 minutes. Consequently it was hypothesized that

vibration may affect grip force by causing hand-tool operators to incorrectly perceive their exerted force levels.

Using the same vibrating hand-tool simulator as in the previous study, subjects held the vibrating handle weighing 15 N for 30 min using a 30:30 s work: rest duty cycle.[99] The handle was vibrating at 8 m/s² ISO weighted acceleration[100], for frequencies of 20 Hz, 80 Hz, and 160 Hz, in three orthogonal directions. Immediately following exposure, index finger ridge height detection sensory thresholds were determined using an apparatus designed after Corlett et al.[101] Average falling ridge thresholds increased 0.01 mm (50 percent) at 20 Hz and 80 Hz, and increased 0.03 mm (150 percent) at 160 Hz. No significant rising ridge thresholds were observed, however. Since tactility decreased with increasing frequency between 20 Hz and 160 Hz, it was concluded that loss of tactility was not likely to be the cause of increased grip force since grip force was greatest at the low-frequency (40 Hz) vibration.

Based on these results, it is recommended that tasks requiring a high degree of tactile sensitivity, such as inspecting for smoothness or rough edges, should avoid involving tools producing vibration in the 160 Hz range since sensory performance, and thus work performance in manual inspection tasks, may be affected. Sanding and grinding operations are two examples. Workers often sand or grind a surface and periodically inspect their work using tactile inspection to determine if the surface is sanded to the desired level of smoothness. Diminished tactility may result in a surface feeling smoother than it actually is, resulting in a rougher surface than actually desired.

EVALUATION AND CONTROL OF ERGONOMIC STRESSES

There are no particular guidelines or standards indicating acceptable exposure limits for combined vibration and ergonomic stress factors to prevent chronic muscle and nerve problems. The ISO 5349 "Hand and Arm Vibration Exposure Standard" [102] emphasizes the vascular effects of HAV. As yet there are no vibration standards for protecting workers from neuromuscular CTDs, localized muscle fatigue, or for controlling manual performance deficits caused from exposure to HAV. Hence the best approach is to minimize these stress factors.

Although previous studies have shown that CTDs are associated with repetitive motions, forceful exertions, contact stresses, postural stresses, low temperatures, and vibration, there is no consensus among researchers about what levels, either alone or in combination with other factors, can be safely tolerated. As a result, problem situations are often identified *after* workers have been affected. In these situations epidemiological methods may be employed to evaluate the morbidity pattern to identify specific work areas, jobs, and tools with elevated risk.[103,104] Morbidity patterns may be determined from available data (first aid reports, workers' compensation reports, and OSHA records), or from health surveys where workers are interviewed or given physical examinations. In some cases localized fatigue may be used as an indicator of possible CTDs and to identify stressful jobs. Experience has shown that these disorders often go unreported and that more cases are found through interviews and physical examinations than through plant medical department visits and compensation reports.

Job analysis is used to identify specific work factors that might be causing the problem. These factors may be modified through work station, tool, material, process, and method changes to alleviate the injury and illness patterns. Since safe levels are not yet known, they should be evaluated to ascertain their effectiveness. Available morbidity studies suggest that nearly all hand-intensive jobs have some potential for producing CTDs in workers. As a result, employers should be vigilant and search for such disorders and not wait for worker complaints before analyzing their health data and jobs.

Job analysis entails (1) documenting the job, and (2) assessing the major ergonomic stresses associated with CTDs, (vibration exposure, repetitiveness, forcefulness, contact stresses and postural stresses). Because the same principals are used in evaluation as are used in control, these steps will be considered together.

The purpose of documentation is to collect the data needed to perform an assessment of ergonomic stresses and to design interventions. Also, the documentation serves as a permanent record of how the job was performed at the time of the analysis. The documentation entails determining and recording job-specific attributes. The job attributes can be thought of as independent variables. They include: (1) job objective, (2) work standard, (3) staffing, (4) workplace layout, (5) tools, (6) materials, (7) personal protective equipment, and (8) methods.

Sources of information for job documentation include: (1) personnel department job descriptions and classifications, (2) industrial engineering department standards and descriptions, (3) supervisors, (4) production and plant engineers, (5) plant drawings, and (6) workers. It is always desirable that the workplace and job be inspected to verify the documentation. Videotapes and still photographs can be used to facilitate documentation.

Once documentation of the job-specific attributes is complete, the ergonomic attributes, repetitiveness, forcefulness, posture, contact stresses, low temperature, and vibration can be considered. Ergonomic attributes and stresses may be thought of as dependent variables in the analysis.

Repetitiveness

Repetitiveness can be calculated from the work standard, staffing, and work method. For example, a work standard may specify removing three rough edges on 1,200 parts per hour. From the staffing information it is determined that this job is performed by six workers. From the methods information it is found that, on the average, the workers must grind three edges. Repetitiveness can then be calculated as:

1,200parts/hr / 6 workers $\times$ 3 exertions / part = 600 exertions / worker / hr

In another situation in which workers use power sanders, it is found that they hold the sander continuously while they sand table tops. Workers sand 16 tables per shift, per worker. The repetitiveness of this job might be better expressed in terms of the duration of the exertions or 480 min/16 = 30 minutes. These values provide reference points for evaluating intervention strategies.

Changing the standard to reduce repetitiveness may raise direct labor cost; however, these costs may be offset by reductions in worker suffering, lost work, and compensation costs. Interventions for repetitiveness include: (1) changing work standards to require fewer exertions per unit time, (2) use of mechanical devices to perform exertions (see Figure 8-8), (3) quality control/maintenance to reduce the number of motions required for surface finishing or redriving defective screws, (4) worker rotations to alternate work loads between different parts of the body, and (5) combining jobs to increase the variety of exertions.

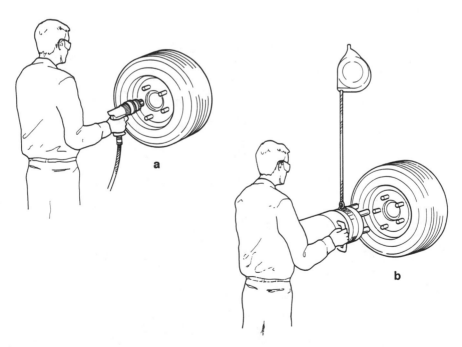

FIGURE 8-8.   The number of exertions and torque loads required for driving studs with a powered nut runner (a) can be reduced using a multiple spindle nut runner (b).

Forcefulness

Force of exertion is related to the load supported or resisted with the hand, the friction between the load and hand, and the posture of the hand.[105-107] The minimum required pinch force can be estimated based on the load and coefficient of friction, however it has been shown that most people will exert more than the minimum, especially for low exertion levels.[108] It suffices to say that as the load increases or the friction decreases, the object must be gripped tighter and greater forces will be transferred to the musculoskeletal system. This principal can be used to both assess job strength requirements and for designing the job to minimize strength requirements. Interventions for forcefulness include increasing friction or decreasing load.

Steps for increasing friction include use of high-friction surface materials and textures in handle design,[109,110] and high-friction materials for glove design.[111] Steps for decreasing load include: (1) use of lightweight tools, (2) use of hoists and articulating arms for supporting heavy tools[112] (see Figure 8-9), (3) balancing tools around the center of grip (see Figure 8-10), (4) use of torque-control devices, (5) tools that stop at specified torque settings, (6) multiple spindle nut runners (see Figure 8-8), (7) reaction bars (see Figure 8-9), (8) selection of well-fitting gloves,[113]

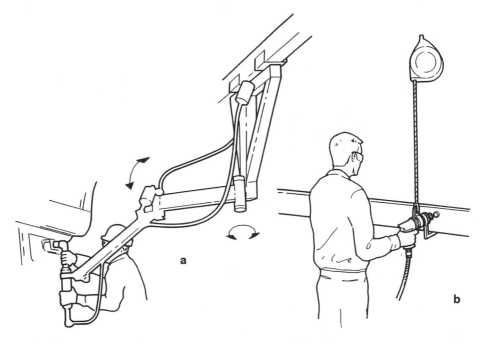

FIGURE 8-9.   Articulating arms, and hoists can be used to reduce the weight and torque forces associated with power tools (a). A torque reaction bar sometimes can be used to transfer loads back to the work piece (b). Special attention may be required to install torque reaction bars so that minimal effort is required to hold and use the tools in the work position.

(9) selection of fasteners that minimize force to engage bits, (10) use of a quality control program to minimize force required to fit parts, and (11) maintaining equipment, such as screwdrivers, to avoid forces associated with worn bits and excessive torque settings[114]

The loads in the musculoskeletal system will also be affected by the posture of the hand. The muscles have to work harder if the objects are pinched than if they are held in a power grip[115,116]. Possible interventions for forceful exertions should also include design of handles so that they can be held in a power or hook grip posture (see Figure 8-11).

Posture

While it is not desirable to immobilize the body in one ideal posture, some postures are more stressful than others. As a general rule, it is desirable to keep the elbow at the side of the body, to avoid extreme rotation of the forearm, to avoid extreme deviation of the wrist side to side, to avoid wrist flexion (toward the palm of the hand), or extreme wrist extension (toward the back of the hand) (see Figure 8-1). Posture is related to work location, work position, tool shape, and worker size. Posture interventions include: (1) relocation of work, (2) reorientation of work, and (3) selection of an alternative tool design (see Figure 8-12).

The location, orientation, and tool design must all be considered together along with the stature of the worker.[117, 118] In situations where the work location and orientation cannot be adjusted to suit the worker, it may be possible to select another tool. In cases where the work specifications determine the tool design, it may be possible to change the location or orientation. It is possible to estimate the ideal work location for a given worker and tool. Figure 8-13 shows how the ideal work height can be estimated for a worker using an in-line screwdriver on a horizontal surface as the elbow height minus the tool height. Figure 8-13 also shows how the ideal height for a worker using a pistol grip screwdriver on a vertical surface as elbow height plus tool height.

Where possible, the location and orientation for a given tool should be adjustable to accommodate workers of different sizes. The range of adjustability can be estimated for a given rage of the population using link-length data and anatomical mannequins. Figure 8-14 shows the major body segments expressed as a fraction of stature. Average segment lengths for a given stature can be estimated by multiplying the segment fraction times stature.[119] Figure 8-15 shows how link-length data were used to estimate the desired work heights for an in-line screwdriver on a horizontal work surface for persons between 5th percentile female and 95th percentile male statures, 151.1 cm and 186.9 cm, respectfully.[120] Ideally the work should be adjustable between these extremes. Although two-dimensional analysis is adequate for many work situations, it is sometimes necessary to extend it to three

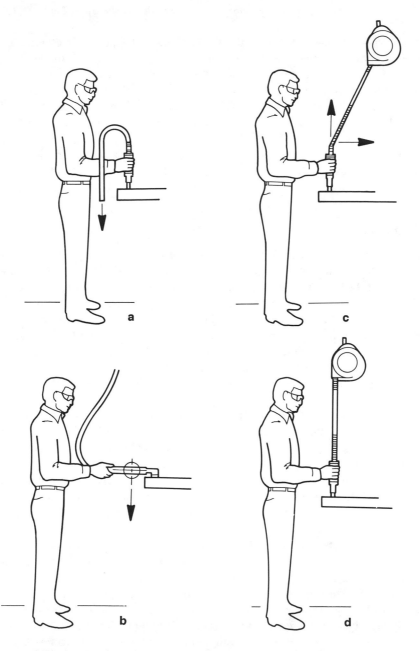

FIGURE 8-10. Forcefulness may be adversely affected by the additional weight of pneumatic tool air hoses (a). These forces can be reduced by relocating handles or airline attachments (b) or use of counterbalancers. Special attention may be required to be sure that the balancer is attached directly above the work as in (d) and not in (c).

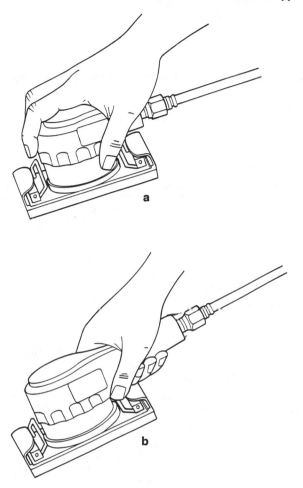

FIGURE 8-11.   Handles that require pinch grip postures should be avoided (a). Handles should be designed so that they can be held in a power grip posture (b).

dimensions. Figure 8-14b shows how the length on a shoulder link can be adjusted for abduction of the shoulder (movement away from the side of the body).

Drawing board, mannequins are silhouettes of the body that can be positioned on a drawing to determine required posture and reach capability.[121, 122] It is now possible to digitize the mannequin segments and perform a posture and reach analysis using microcomputers.[123]

In all cases, theoretical predictions should be verified by observing experienced workers performing similar jobs. It is important that workers observed be representative of the statures and gender for the intended work force.

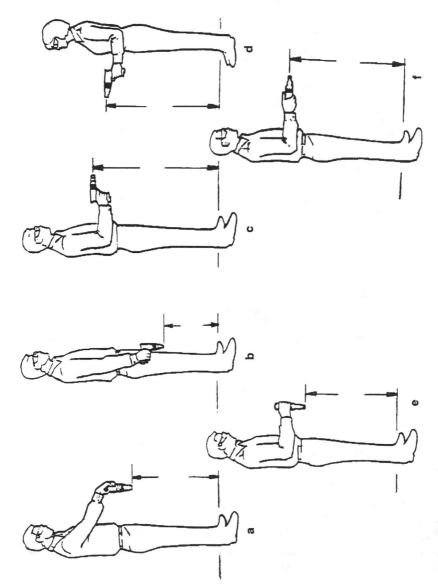

FIGURE 8-12. Use of a pistol grip power tool on a horizontal surface (a) may result in stressful work postures. Interventions may include: relocation of work (b), reorientation of work considering anthropometric characteristics of workers (c and d), or selection of alternative tool handle designs (e). Similarly, stressful posture from use of an in-line power tool on a vertical surface (f) may be eliminated by reorienting the work (e).

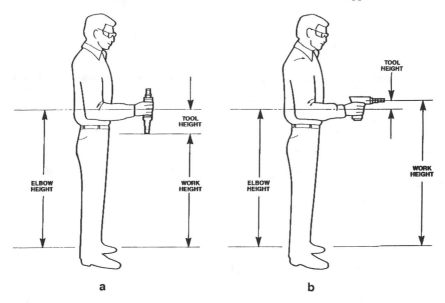

FIGURE 8-13. The ideal work height for a worker using an in-line tool on a horizontal surface is estimated as the elbow height minus the tool height (a). The ideal height for a worker using a pistol grip hand tool on a vertical surface is estimated as the elbow height plus the tool height (b).

Contact Stress

Contact stress is produced when the body comes in contact with external objects. Examples include leaning on the elbows, resting the forearm and wrist on sharp edges of benches, tools that are supported over the base of the palm or rubbed on the sides of the fingers (see Figure 8-16). Contact stress interventions include: (1) reducing the required force to hold and use a tool by the previous methods suggested, (2) eliminating sharp edges from triggers and handles that might produce a stress concentration[124, 125] (see Figure 8-16), (3) lengthening handles to eliminate contact with sharp edges (see Figure 8-16), and providing gloves or pads when sharp edges cannot be eliminated.

Low Temperature

Skin temperatures below 75° F may have an adverse effect on manipulative ability and increase the risk of CTDs. Reduced skin temperatures may result from lowered body temperatures, exposure to cold ambient or tool exhaust air, or contact with cold parts and materials. Intervention strategies for lowered skin temperatures include: (1) use of clothing to retain body heat, (2) use of gloves to retain extremity blood flow and heat, (3) increased air temperature to reduce convective heat loss

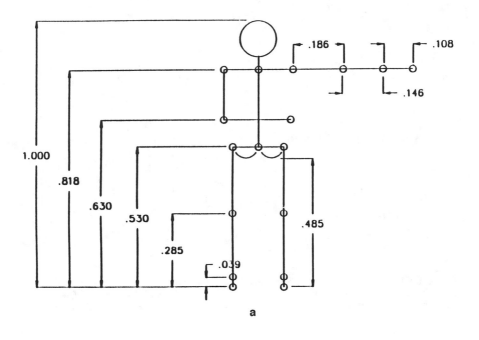

a

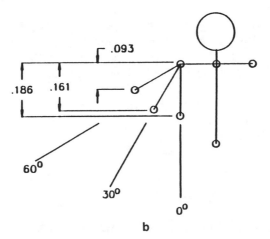

b

FIGURE 8-14. Link fractions are multiplied by stature to estimate average link lengths (a). Upper arm link lengths may be adjusted for reaches outside of the saggittal plane (b).

144

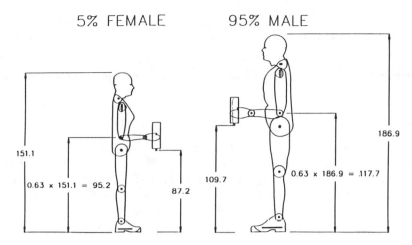

FIGURE 8-15.   Work height should be adjustable to accommodate 5th percentile female to a 95th percentile male.

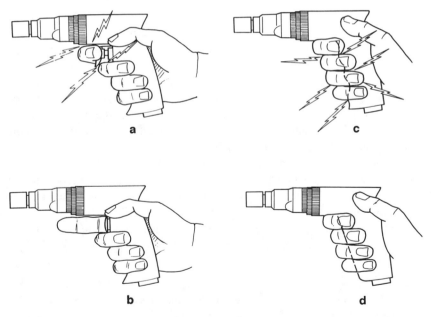

FIGURE 8-16.   Contact stress from prolonged contact with sharp tool trigger edges (a), can be reduced by using rounded smooth surfaces for redistributing the forces (b). Tool handles with indentations for fingers should be avoided (c) because they don't always fit in the hand as intended and contact with protruding surfaces can concentrate forces at the volar surfaces of the fingers. Use of a smooth handle surface can avoid this problem (d).

145

from the body, (4) directing exhaust air away from the hand to prevent heat loss, (5) warming parts and materials to warm the hand or at least prevent conductive losses, and (6) use of low thermal conductive materials for handles to prevent conductive losses.

Vibration

Some tool manufacturers are now offering tools designed to produce less vibration.[126] Add-on accessories for standard tool handles have been met so far with mixed success. Although rubber handle coverings did not significantly reduce vibration, Radwin and Armstrong[127] found their use resulted in lower grip exertions. This may be due to improved frictional characteristics between the hands and tool handle. Personal protection devices such as antivibration gloves are another method of providing vibration isolation to the hands and arms. A problem with some antivibration gloves is the large amount of absorbing material necessary, making grasp difficult and interfering with hand motions. Even if gloves or other antivibriation apparel can prevent vibration transmission to the hands, they should be used cautiously. Gloves may increase grip exertions, especially poorly fitting gloves.

SUMMARY

Ergonomic factors such as repetitiveness, forcefulness, contact stress, posture, low temperature, in addition to vibration can cause, precipitate, and aggravate upper extremity nerve disorders such as CTS. Since these factors usually occur together, it is inadequate to deal only with vibration, and all of the aforementioned ergonomic stress factors must be addressed together.

Vibration may increase the risk of CTDs as a result of excessive force exerted when holding some vibrating hand tools. The studies described here have dealt with short-term effects of vibration exposure. It is reasonable to expect, however, that these short-term effects observed can lead to long-term disabilities. The impact of these effects ultimately on health are not yet known. That is to say it is not known how much grip force can be exerted without excessive risk of incurring CTDs.

Notes

1. Taylor, W. and Pelmear, P. L. *Vibration White Finger in Industry*. London: Academic Press, 1975:166.
2. Brammer, A. J. and Taylor, W. *Vibration Effects on the Hand and Arm in Industry*. John Wiley & Sons, 1982.
3. Brammer, A. J. *Exposure of the Hand to Vibration in Industry*. Ottawa, Canada: Environment Secretariat, 1984; NRCC Publication No. 22844.

4. Kumlin, T.; Wikeri, M.; Sumari, P. Radiological Changes in Carpal and Metacarpal Bones and Phalanges Caused by Chain Saw Vibration. *British Journal of Industrial Medicine* 1973; 30:71–73.
5. Gemne, G. and Taylor, W. *Hand-Arm Vibration and the Central Autonomic Nervous System.* London: Multi-Science Publishing Co., Ltd., 1983.
6. Miwa, T. "Evaluation Methods for Vibration Effect: Part 3: Measurements of Threshold and Equal Sensation Countours on Hand for Vertical and Horizontal Sinusoudal Vibrations. *Industrial Health* 1967; 5:213–220.
7. Mishoe, J. W. and Suggs, C.W. Hand-Arm Vibration. Part I: Subjective Response to Single and Multi-Directional Sinusoidal and Non-Sinusoidal Excitation. *Journal of Sound and Vibration* 1974; 35(4):479–488.
8. Miwa, T. "Evaluation Methods for Vibration Effect: Part 6. Measurements of Unpleasant and Tolerance Limit Levels for Sinusoidal Vibrations. *Industrial Health* 1968; 6:18–27.
9. Hasan, J. "Biomedical Aspects of Low-Frequency Vibration: A Selective Review." *Work-Environment-Health* 1970; 6(1):19–45.
10. Rothfleisch, S. and Sherman, D. "Carpal Tunnel Syndrome: Biomechanical Aspects of Occupational Occurrence and Implications Regarding Surgical Management. *Orthopaedic Review* 1978; 7:107–109.
11. Lukas, E. Lesion of the Peripheral Nervous System due to Vibration. *Work-Environment-Health* 1970; 7(1):67–79.
12. Brammer, *Exposure of the Hand.*
13. Lukas, "Lesion of the Peripheral Nervous System."
14. Cannon, L. J.; Bernacki, E. J.; Walter, S. D.; "Personal and Occupational Factors Associated With Carpal Tunnel Syndrome." *Journal of Occupational Medicine* 1981; 23:255–258.
15. Seppalainen, A. M. "Nerve Conduction in the Vibration Syndrome." *Scandinavian Journal of Work, Environment-Health* 1970; 7:82–84.
16. Rothfleisch and Sherman. "Carpal Tunnel Syndrome."
17. Cannon, Bernacki, and Walter, "Personal and Occupational Factors."
18. Silverstein, B. A. Armstrong, T. J. Fine L. J. "Hand Wrist Cumulative Trauma Disorders in Industry." *British Journal of Industrial Medicine* 1986; 43:779–784.
19. Silverstein, B. A. Fine, L. J. Armstrong, T. J. "Occupational Factors and Carpal Tunnel Syndrome." *American Journal of Industrial Medicine* 1987; 11: 340–358.
20. Obolenskaja, A. J. and Goljanitzki, I. A., "Die seröse tendo vaginitis in der klinik und im experiment." Dtsch. Z. Chir. 1927; 201:388–399.
21. Hammer. A. W. "Tenosynovitis". *Medical Records* 1934; 140:353–355.
22. Tichauer, E. R. "Some Aspects of Stress on Forearm and Hand in Industry." *Journal of Occupational Medicine* 1966; 8:63–71.
23. Luopajarvi, T.; Kuorinka, I, Virolainen, M., Holmberg, M. "Prevalence of Tenosynovitis and Other Injuries of the Upper Extremities in Repetitive Work". *Scandinavian Journal of Work-Environment-Health* 1979; 5(Suppl.3): 48–55.
24. Kuorinka, L. and Koskinen, P. "Occupatinal Rheumatic Diseases and Upper Limb Strain in Manual Jobs in a Light Mechanical Industry. *Scandinavian Journal of Work-Environment-Health* 1975; 5(Suppl.3):39–47.
25. Silverstein, Fine, and Armstrong, "Occupational Factors."

26. Luopajarvi, Kuorinka, Virolainen, and Holmberg, "Prevalence of Tensqnoitis."
27. Thompson, A.; Plewes, L.; Shaw, E. Peritendonitis Crepitans and Simple Tenosynovitis: A Clinical Study of 544 Cases in Industry. *British Journal of Industrial Medicine* 1951; 8:150–160.
28. Wilson, R. and Wilson, S. "Tenosynovitis in Industry." *Practitioner* 1957; 178:612–615.
29. Muckart, R. "Stenosing Tendovaginitis of the Abductor Pollicis Longus and Extensor Pollicis Brevis at the Radial Styloid (De Quervain's Disease)." *Clinical Orthopaedics* 1964; 33:201–208.
30. Welch, R. "The Causes of Tenosynovitis in Industry." *Industrial Medicine* 1972; 41:16–19.
31. Armstrong, T. J. and Chaffin, D. B. "Carpal Tunnel Syndrome and Selected Personal Attributes." *Journal of Occupational Medicine* 1979; 21(7):481–486.
32. Silverstein, Fine., and Armstrong. "Occupational Factors."
33. Jensen, T. R.; Radwin, R. G.; Webster, J. G. A Conductive Polymer Sensor for Measuring External Finger Forces. *Journal of Biomechanics* 1991; 24:851–858.
34. Tichauer, Some Aspects of Stress.
35. Thompson, Plewes, and Shawn. "Peritendonitis Crepitans."
36. Brain, W. R.; Wright, A. D. Wilknson. M. "Spontaneous Compression of Both Median Nerves in the Carpal Tunnel." *Lancet* 1947; 1:277–282.
37. Tanzer, R. "The Carpal Tunnel Sydrome." *Journal of Bone and Joint Surgery* 1959; 41A:626–634.
38. Robbins, H. "Anatomical Study of the Median Nerve in the Carpal Tunnel and Etiologies of Carpal Tunnel Syndrome." *Journal of Bone and Joint Surgery* 1963; 45A:953–966.
39. Phalen, G. "The Carpal Tunnel Syndrome." *Journal of Bone and Joint Surgery.*1966; 48A:211–228.
40. Phalen, G. "The Carpal Tunnel Syndrome, Clinical Evaluation of 598 Hands." *Clinical Orthapeadics Related Research* 1972; 83:29–40.
41. Smith, E.; Sonstegard, D.; Anderson, W. "Contribution of Flexor tendons to the Carpal Tunnel Syndrome. *Archives of Physical Medicine & Rehabilitation* 1977; 58:379–385.
42. Lundborg., G.; Gelberman, R. H.; Minetter-Convery, M.; Lee. Y. Hargens, A. R. "Median Nerve Compression in the Carpal Tunnel—functional Reponse to Experimentally Induced Controlled Pressure. *The Journal of Hand Surgery* 1982; 7(3):252–259.
43. Armstrong, T. J.; Castelli, W.; Evans, F. G.; Diaz-Perez, R. Some Histological Changes in the Carpal Tunnel Contents and Their Biomechamical Implications. *Journal of Occupational Medicine* 1984; 26(3):197–201.
44. Tichauer, "Some Aspects of Stress."
45. Thompson, Plewes, and Shaw. "Peritendonotis Crepitans."
46. Armstrong and Chaffin, "Carpal Tunnel Syndrome."
47. Gray, H. *Classic Collector's Edition: Gray's Anatomy.* New York: Bounty Books, 1977.
48. Stein, A. H.; Ramsey, R. H.; Key, J. A. "Stenosing Tenovaginitis at the Radiostyloid Process (De Quervain's Disease)." *Archives of Surgery* 1951; 63:216–228.

49. Younghusband, O. and Black, J. "De Quervain's Disease: Stenosing Tenovaginitis at the Radial Styloid Process." *Canadian Medical Association Journal* 1963; 89:508–512.
50. Kelley, A. and Jacobson, H. "Hand Disability due to Tenosynovitis." *Industrial Medicine and Surgery* 1964: 570–574.
51. Lamphier, T.; Crooker, C. Crooker, J.; "De Quervain's Disease." *Industrial Medicine and Surgery* 1965; 34:847–856.
52. Tichauer, E. R. "Biomechanics Sustains Occupational Safety and Health." *Industrial Engineering* 1976 (Feb):46–56.
53. Hoffman, G. "Tendonitis and burtisis." *American Family Practice* 1981; 23:103–110.
54. Kurppaawarisa, Rokkanen, "Tennis Elbow."
55. Hoffman, "Tendonitis and Bursitis."
56. Goldie, I. "Epicondylitis Lateralis Humeri: Apathogentical Study." *Acta Chirurgica Scandinavica* 1964(suppl. 339):119.
57. Bora, F. and Osterman, A. "Compression Neuropathy." *Clinical Orthopaedics* 1982; 163:20–31.
58. Feldman, R.; Goldman, R. Keyserling, W. M.; "Peripheral Nerve Entrapment Syndromes and Ergonomics Factors." *American Journal of Industrial Medicine* 1983; 4:6–11.
59. MacNicol, M. "Extraneural Pressures Affecting Ulnar Nerve at the Elbow." *Hand* 1982; 14:6–11.
60. Pechan, J. and Julis I. "The Pressure Measurement in the Ulnar Nerve: A Contribution to the Pathophysiology of the Cubital Tunnel Syndrome." *Journal of Biomechanics* 1975; 8:75–79.
61. Spans, F. "Occupational Nerve Lesions." In: Vinken, P. and Bruyn, G. eds. *Handbook of Clinical Neurology*. New York: Elsevier, 1970; 7:326–343.
62. Wadsworth, T.; Williams, J. "Cubital Tunnel Compression Syndrome." *British Medical Journal* 1973; 1:662–666.
63. Kisner, "Thumb Neuroma: A Hazard of Ten Pin Bowling." *British Journal of Plastic Surgery* 1976; 29:225–226.
64. Dobyns, J. H.; O'Brien, E. T.; Linscheid, R. L.; Farrow, G.M. "Bowler's Thumb: Diagnosis and Treatment." *The Journal of Bone and Joint Surgery* 1972; 54A(4):751–755.
65. Sperling, W. "Snapping Finger: Roentgen Treatment and Experimental Production." *Acta. Radiology* 1951; 37:74–80.
66. Quinnel, R. "Conservative Management of Trigger Finger." *Practitioner* 1980; 224:187–190.
67. Tichauer, "Some Aspects of Stress."
68. Phalen, "The Carpal-Tunnel Syndrome."
69. Kendall, D. "Aetiology, Diagnosis and Treatment of Paraesthesia in Hands." *British Medical Journal* 1960; 2:1633–1640.
70. Hoffman, J. and Hoffman, P. L. "Staple Gun Carpal Tunnel Syndrome." *Journal of Occupational Medicine* 1985; 27(11):848–849.
71. Szabo, R. M. and Gelberman, R. H. "The Pathophysiology of Nerve Entrapment Syndromes." *Journal of Hand Surgery* 1987; 12A(5)(Part2):880–884.

72. Clark, R. "The limiting hand skin temperature Unaffected Manual Performance in the Cold." *Journal of Applied Psychology* 1961; 45:193-194.
73. Dusek, R. "Effect of Temperature on Manual Performance." In: Fisher, R., ed. *Production and Functioning of the Hands in Cold Climates.* Washington, DC: National Academy of Sciences, National Research Council, 1957:63-76.
74. Fox, W. "Human Performance in the Cold." *Human Factors* 1967; 9:203-220.
75. Lockhart, J. and Kiess, H. "Auxiliary Heating of the Hands During Cold Exposure and Manual Performance." *Human Factors* 1071; 13:457-465.
76. Mackworth, N. "Cold Acclimatization and Finger Numbness." *Proceedings of the Royal Society* 1955; 143:392-404.
77. Morton, R. and Provins, K. "Finger Numbness After Acute Local Exposure to Cold." *Journal of Applied Physiology* 1960; 15:149-154.
78. Georgitis, J. "Extensor Tenosynovitis of the Hand From Cold Exposure." *Journal of the Maine Medical Association* 1978; 69:129-131.
79. Wasserman, D. E.; Reynolds, D. D.; Behrens, V.; Taylor, W.; Samueloff, S. *Vibration White Finger Disease in U.S. Workers Using Pneumatic Chipping and Grinding Hand Tools.* Cincinnati, OH: NIOSH, 1981; DHHS Publication No. 82-101.
80. National Institute for Occupational Safety and Health. "Vibration Syndrome in Chipping and Grinding Workers." *Journal of Occupational Medicine* 1984; 26(Suppl. 10):765-788.
81. Radwin, R. G. and Armstrong, T. J. "Assessment of Hand Vibration Exposure on an Assembly Line." *American Industrial Hygiene Association Journal* 1985; 46(4):211-219.
82. Pyykko, I.; Farkkila, M.; Toivanen, J.; Korhonen, O.; Hyvarinen, J. "Transmission of Vibration in the Hand-Arm System With Special References to Changes in Compression Force and Acceleration." *Scandinavian Journal of Work-Environment-Health* 1976; 2:87-95.
83. Iwata, H. Dupuis, H. Hartung, E. "Ubertrang von horizontalen sinusschwingungen auf die oberen extremitaten bei halbpronationsstellung und reaktion des m. biceps." *Int. Arch. Arbeitsmed* 1972; 30:313-328.
84. Reynolds, D. D. "Hand-Arm Vibration: A Review of 3 Years' Research." In: Wasserman, D. E. and Taylor, W, eds. *Proceedings of the International Occupational Hand-Arm Vibration Conference.* Cincinnati: U.S. Department of Health Education, and Welfare, 1977: 99-128 (DHEW Publication No. 77-170).
85. Brammer, A. J.; Taylor, W.; Lundborg, G. "Sesorineural Signs of the Hand-Arm Vibration Syndrome." *Scandinavian Journal of Work-Environment, and Health.* 1987; 13:279-283.
86. Lukas, "Lesion of the Periphereal Nervous System."
87. Radwin, R. G. "Neuromuscular Effects of Vibrating Hand Tools on Grip Exertions, Tactility, Discomfort, and Fatigue (Dissertation)." Ann Arbor, MI: The University of Michigan, 1986.
88. Radwin, R. G.; Armstrong, T. J.; Chaffin, D. B. "Power Hand Tool Vibration Effects on Grip Exertions." *Ergonomics* 1987; 30(5):833-855.
89. Rood O. N. "On Contraction of the Muscles Induced by Contact With Bodies in Vibration." *American Journal of Science* 1860; 29(87):449.

90. Matthews, P. B. C. "The Reflex Excitation of the Soleus Muscle of the Decrebrate Cat Caused by Vibration Applied to Its Tendon." *Journal of Physiology* 1966; 184:450–472.
91. Hagbarth, E. and Eklund, G. "Motor Effects of Vibratory Muscle Stimuli in Man." In: Granit, R., ed. *Muscular Afferents and Motor Control.* New York: John Wiley & Sons, 1965:177–186.
92. Lance, J. W.; De Gail, P.; Neilson, P. D.; "Tonic and Phasic Spinal Cord Mechanisms in Man." *Journal of Neurology, Neurosurgery and Psychiatry* 1966; 29:535–544.
93. Radwin, *Neuromuscular Effects.*.
94. International Organization for Standardization (ISO). *Guidelines for the Measurement and Assessment of Human Exposure to Hand-Transmitted Vibration.* International Standard ISO/DIS 5349, 1986.
95. Westling, G. and Johansson, R. S. "Factors Influencing the Force Control During Precision Grip." *Experimental Brain Research* 1984; 53:277–284.
96. Rood, "On Contraction."
97. Streeter, H. "Effects of Localized Vibration on the Human Tactile Sense." *American Industrial Hygiene Association Journal* 1970; 31:87–91.
98. Kume, Y.; Maeda, S.; Hashimoto, F. "Effect of Localized Vibration in Work Environment on Organic Functions at Finger Tip for Surface Roughness." In: *Proceedings of the 1984 International Conference on Occupational Ergonomics.* Redale, ON: Human Factors Society of Canada, 1984:457–461.
99. Radwin, *Neuromuscular Effects.*
100. ISO, *Guidelines.*
101. Corlett, E. N.; Akinmayowa, N. K.; Sivayoganathan, K. "A New Aesthesiometer for Investigating Vibration White Finger (VWF)." *Ergonomics* 1981; 24(1):49–54.
102. ISO, *Guidelines.*
103. Silverstein, Fine, and Armstong., "Occupation Factors."
104. Monson, R. R. *Occupational Epidemiology.* Boca Raton: CRC Press, 1980.
105. Westling and Johansson, "Factors Influencing the Force Control."
106. Armstrong, T. J. "Mechanical Considerations of the Skin in Work." *American Journal of Industrial Medicine* 1985; 87:463–472.
107. Buchholz, B.; Frederick, L. J.; Armstrong T. J. "An Investigation of Human Palmar Skin Friction and the Effects of Materials, Pinch Force and Moisture." *Erigonomics* 1987; 31(3):317–325.
108. Westling and Johansson, "Factors Influencing the Force Control."
109. Buchholz, Frederick, and Armstrong, "An Investigation of Human Palmar Skin."
110. Bobjer, O. "Screwdriver Handles—Design for Power and Precision." *Proceedings of the 1984 International Conference on Occupational Ergonomics* 1984:443–446.
111. Cochran, D. and Riley, M.W. "The Effects of Handle Shape and Size on Exerted Forces." *Human Factors* 1986; 28:253–266.
112. VanBergeijk, E. "Selection of Power Tools and Mechanical Assists for Control of Occupational Hand and Wrist Injuries." *Ergonomic Interventions to Prevent Musculoskeletal Injuries in Industry.* Chelsea, MI: Lewis Publishers, 1987:151–160.
113. Hertzberg, T. "Some Contributions of Applied Physical Anthropometry to Human Engineering." *Annals of the New York Academy of Sciences* 1955; 63(4):616–629.
114. Nenzen, B. "Worn Tools: Another Cause of Injury." *Working Environment*: 1987: 22–23(Sweden).

115. Lundborg, Gelberman, Minteer-Convery, Lee, and Hargens, "Median Nerve Compression."

116. Chao, E.; Opgrande, J.; Axmear, F. "Three-Dimensional Force Analysis of Finger Joints in Selected Isometric Hand Functions." *Journal of Biomechanics* 1976; 9:387–396.

117. Armstrong, T. J.; Radwin., R. G.; Hansen, D. J.; Kennedy, W. "Repetitive Trauma Disorders: Job Evaluation and Design." *Human Factors* 1986; 28(3):325–336.

118. Armstrong, T. J. "Ergonomics and Cumulative Trauma Disorders." *Hand Clinics* 1986; 2(3):553–565.

119. Drillis, R. and Contini, R. "Body Segment Parameters." New York University: Office of Vocational Rehabilitation, Department of Health, Education and Welfare, 1966; Report No. 1166-03.

120. USDHEW. "Weight and Height of Adults 18–74 Years of Age: United States 1971–74." Hyattsville, MD: U.S. Department of Health, Education and Welfare, Public Health Service, Office of Health Research, Statistics and Technology, 1979; Vital and Health Statistics Series, No. 211.

121. Dempster, W. "Space Requirements of the Seated Operator: Geometrical, Kinematic, and Mechanical Aspects of the Body with Special Reference to the Limbs. WADC Technical Report No. 55-159, 1955.

122. Kennedy, K. *Reach Capability of Men and Women: A Three Dimensional Analysis.* Ohio: Wright Patterson Air Force Base, 1978; AMRL-TR-77-50.

123. Armstrong, Radwin., Hansen, and Kennedy, "Repetitive Trauma Disorders."

124. Hoffman, "Tendonitis and Bursitis."

125. Grenberg. L. and Chaffin, D. B. *Workers and Their Tools.* Midland, MI: Pendell Publishers Press, 1976.

126. Yamawaki, S. "Reduction of Vibration in Power Saws in Japan." *Proceedings of the International Occupational Hand-Arm Vibration Conference* 1977:209-217(DHEW (NIOSH) Publication No.77-170).

127. Radwin, R. G. and Armstrong, T. J. A *Study of Physical Stresses Associated with Pneumatic Screwdrivers (Technical Report).* Ann Arbor, MI: The University of Michigan Center for Ergonomics, 1982.

9

Measurements and Basic Principles of Hand-Arm Vibration

D. E. Wasserman

In many ways the measurements of vibration on the human hand are similar to other well-known measurements such as electrocardiograms (ECGs) or electromyograms (EMGs), using surface-mounted electrodes. In ECG measurements, we measure minute electrical potentials generated by the heart. In EMG measurements, we observe the minute electrical firings of muscle fibers. Both of these measurements result from internally generated electrical signals within the human body and radiate to the body surface where they are detected and amplified. In the case of hand-arm vibration (HAV) measurements, the vibration is externally generated from a vibrating hand tool, thus we measure either the vibration motion on the tool itself or at the third metacarpal of the hand. The latter is the resulting motion response of the hand to externally generated vibration; the former is the maximum vibration-tool hazard available to the worker. However, unlike ECGs and EMGs, this mechanical vibratory motion must first be measured, then converted into corresponding minute electrical signals, and finally amplified and stored in order to be useful.

VIBRATION MEASUREMENT COORDINATE SYSTEMS

Vibration is a vector quantity. In order to describe this vibration motion we must know *both* the direction *and* the intensity (magnitude) of the vibration. But the vibration motion at any one point on the hand can move in many ways: up and down, back and forth, or side to side. For simplicity, this "linear" motion can be viewed as moving in three mutually perpendicular directions or axes. Around each of these axes, "rotational" motion can occur, these are called "pitch, yaw, and roll." Thus there are up to three linear motions and three rotational motions at any given

153

single measurement point on the body. For simplicity we measure only the linear motion in each of these three axes.

In order to compare HAV measurements worldwide, a series of biodynamic/basicentric coordinate systems are used and are shown in Figure 9-1. It is usually easier to measure vibration on tool handles nearest where the worker grasps the tool (basicentric system). Figure. 9-2 shows the actual use of this system and the corresponding placement and orientation of three perpendicular vibration transducers on the handles of a grinder, located where the operator grips the tool. When making these measurements, vibration transducers should all be as light as possible ("flyweight") to avoid errors. If the biodynamic system is used, then three mutually perpendicular transducers are mounted noninvasively on the hand. An alcohol scrub is used to clean the skin surface at the third metacarpal followed by stiff carpet tape, which is then placed between the skin surface and the transducers per Figure 9-3.[1]

BASIC PRINCIPLES

When we speak of vibratory motion, we usually refer to motion of an object starting at some reference point and then moving off to another position in either of the three linear directions (and/or rotational directions). The distance the object has traversed is called *displacement*. The units of displacement are given as meters, millimeters, centimeters, inches, and feet. It obviously took some time for the object to move from its initial position to its new position. If we in effect divide the distance traversed by this time factor, we get the *speed or velocity* of the moving object. More precisely, velocity is the time rate of change of displacement. The

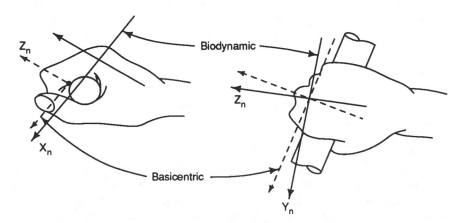

FIGURE 9-1.   Basicentric and biodynamic coordinate systems used for hand-tool and hand-arm vibration measurements. (Courtesy ACGIH)

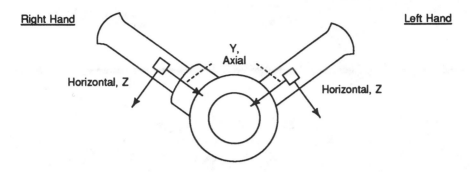

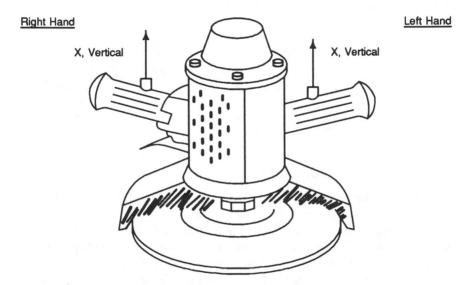

FIGURE 9-2.   Use of basicentric coordinate system and accelerometer placements to measure grinder vibration. (Adapted from Wasserman et al., "Vibration White Finger.")

units of velocity are a ratio of distance to time (for example, ft/sec, in/sec, m/sec, cm/sec, mm/sec).

In many instances the speed of a moving object changes. This time rate of change of speed or velocity is called *acceleration*. The units of acceleration are distance/time/time or m/sec./sec. or ft./sec./sec. It is convenient to compare vibration acceleration to gravitational forces or g where 1 g = 9.81 m/sec./sec. Thus displacement, velocity, and acceleration are three motion units that are all mathematically linked.

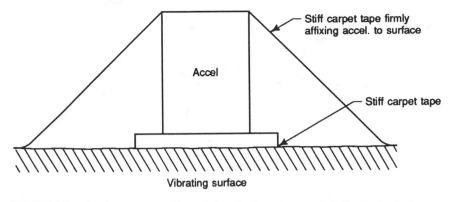

FIGURE 9-3.   Accelerometer mounting technique for the measurement of vibration impinging on the surface of the human body. (Adapted from Wasserman, *Human Aspects of Occupational Vibration.*)

Another characteristic of motion is that it can repeat itself "periodically" over and over again. One full cycle of motion, completed in one second is the *frequency* of vibration, which used to be called cycles/second. Now, it is called hertz or simply Hz. The motion need not necessarily be periodic; it can be nonperiodic or random. Finally, a reminder, vibration is a vector quantity described by both a magnitude and by a direction.

VIBRATION MEASUREMENTS

A typical generic vibration-measurement system is shown in Figure 9-4, using acceleration as the measurement parameter of choice. It is to be noted that corresponding vibration velocity and displacement levels are easily obtained from such a measurement of acceleration by using electronic integration. What is sought is an "averaged" acceleration called *root-mean-squared or (rms).*

Referring to Figure 9-4, it has been previously shown that to measure acceleration, three perpendicularly mounted (crystal or piezoelectric) accelerometers are required for the X, Y, Z axes. This means that each of these three transducers will need separate conditioning (charge) preamplifiers where each simultaneously amplifies the minute electrical signals coming from their respective accelerometers. These amplified signals are then simultaneously recorded and stored on a multitrack frequency modulated (FM) tape recorder for subsequent computer analysis. A conventional multitrack tape recorder cannot be used since it will tend to modify and distort the actual vibration signals such that the computer data analysis will be faulty. Also, since we are recording dynamic motion in the three perpendicular axes at the same point, it is necessary to record all multiaxis vibration data channels simultaneously. An oscilloscope is used to monitor the vibration signals entering each channel of the FM tape

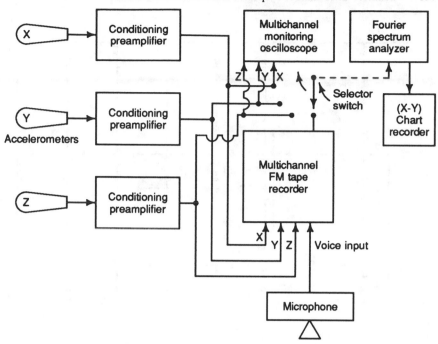

FIGURE 9-4.   A typical triaxial human vibration measurement and data analysis system. (Adapted from Wasserman, reference 7)

recorder to ensure its purity and to avoid equipment overload, which results in an unwanted error called *DC shifting*. A microphone or an electronic time-code generator is usually used to log and later identify the vibration data being recorded. A video camcorder can be useful for identifying motion when used with this system.

VIBRATION DATA ANALYSIS

Computer analysis of vibration data is called Fourier spectrum analysis and seeks to characterize not only the overall vibration (dose) impinging on the body in each of the three directions, but also to characterize the unique spectral characteristics of this vibration by electronically "dissecting" the vibration motion in each direction into its constituent frequency components. An example of Fourier analysis is shown in Figure 9-5 for the Z axis of a vibrating pneumatic chipping hammer,[2] and a typical Fourier graph is shown in Figure 9-6. If we refer to Figure 9-4, we see that the horizontal axis of this spectrum graph displays vibration frequencies from 6.3–1,000 Hz; the vertical axis displays the vibration rms acceleration magnitude or intensity, in m/sec./sec. units, where 1g = 9.81

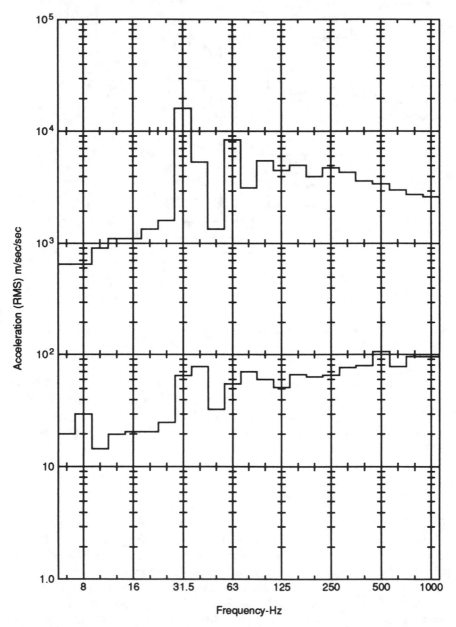

FIGURE 9-5. A Fourier spectrum analysis obtained from a pneumatic chipping hammer used to clean cast iron castings. Chisel spectrum (Top); handle spectrum (Bottom). Both obtained for the axial direction. (Adapted from Wasserman et al., "Vibration White Finger.")

158

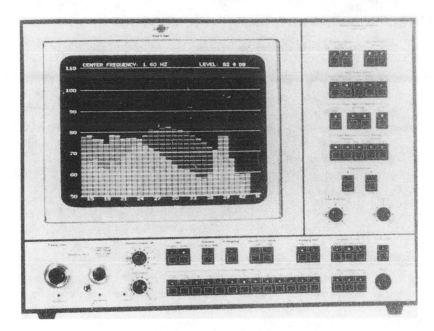

FIGURE 9-6.   A typical Fourier spectrum analyzer. (Courtesy Bruel & Kjaer Co.)

m/sec./sec. There are two spectra shown on the graph. The top spectrum is the vibration measured at the tool's chisel. The bottom spectrum is the vibration in the same axis at the tool handle. Since the vibration spectrum constitutes a unique vibration "fingerprint" of this tool, the top spectrum shows that there is unacceptable overall vibration intensity, with the fundamental vibration frequency impinging on the chisel hand at 31.5 Hz. This fundamental vibration frequency is followed by multiple "harmonics" adding to the overall vibration energy. Many more harmonics (e.g., multiples of the fundamental vibration frequency) can be, and usually are present. Finally, the summation of all these frequency spectra determines the vibration-hazard level the worker receives in that given direction at that measurement point. The bottom spectrum at the tool handle indicates that the overall acceleration at the handle is approximately 200 g (rms), or a significant reduction from that of the chisel hand. This is most likely due to the tool mass and internal damping. In *both* cases, these vibration levels are excessive and unacceptable if we were to compare these values and spectra to existing human hand-arm vibration (HAV) Standards such as the ACGIH-TLV, ANSI S3.34, et cetera. A complete data analysis requires that each vibration axis must be computer analyzed for its spectrum and contribution to the overall vibration impinging on the user's hands.

SIMPLIFIED VIBRATION MEASUREMENTS

The foregoing data analysis provides not only the vibration hazard impinging on the body in each of the three triaxial directions, but it also yields spectral and other data valuable to design engineers, researchers, et cetera. However, Fourier computer analysis can be costly and represent "information overload" to an industrial hygienist, who for example need only refer to existing health and safety standards and merely needs to know vibration-hazard level data in each of the three directions. Portable, commercial instruments are currently available for hand-arm measurements (see Figure 9-7). These will usually provide readouts that must be compared to the appropriate standards. These devices do not provide nor perform a Fourier spectral analysis.

MODELING

To understand and predict the biodynamic effects of vibration impinging on the human body, several engineering "models" have been devised for HAV.[3] These engineering models consist of three elements: mass, springs, and damping elements. The relative arrangement and interconnections of these elements depend not only on the so-called mathmatical "equations of motion" of the system being modeled, but also on the actual physical structure of the human hand. All models are subject to limited assumptions upon which the model is based. Thus their usefulness and accuracy is limited.

HUMAN RESONANCES

One of the very significant and useful contributions of early modeling and measurements research was the discovery of resonances associated with the human body.[4, 5] This concept[6] is best described by giving a well known example. Why is it that soldiers never march in step across a bridge? Instead they break cadence or rhythm and walk across the bridge. If they marched across the bridge in rhythm, the resulting regular, intense low-frequency pounding of their marching would generate vibration excitation of the mechanical bridge structure. The beams of the bridge absorbing this vibration energy and amplifying it. In short order the bridge will begin to sway and eventually collapse. This concept is referred to as *resonance or natural frequency*. At the resonant frequency, the maximum energy transfer from source to receiver occurs. Humans exhibit these same resonance characteristics as do virtually all physical structures, since the human body is composed of mass, spring, and damping elements. It is these elements that determine at what vibration frequencies resonances occur. The concern is that if workers are exposed to HAV containing potentially harmful resonant vibration frequencies, then there is a likelihood that the adverse effects of this exposure would be exacerbated. At

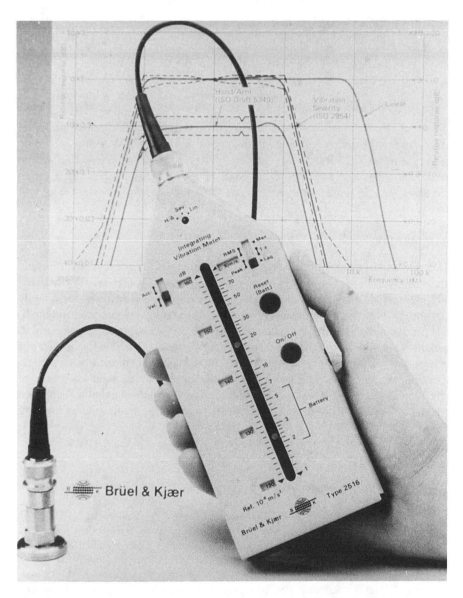

FIGURE 9-7. A typical portable human vibration meter used for hand-arm vibration measurements. (Courtesy Bruel & Kjaer Co.)

161

resonance it takes only a *small* amount of impinging vibration to ellicit a *large* response from a system, whereas at other vibration frequencies it takes a greater amount of impinging vibration to elicit the same response. For HAV, for either of the three linear directions, resonance seems to occur in the 100–250 Hz range.[7, 8] In general, the larger the system mass, the lower the resonant frequency.

One of the reasons for requiring tool-vibration measurements and for performing a Fourier analysis is to determine when, where, and the spectral magnitudes at which these particular vibration frequencies occur. It would appear that resonance is one of the Achilles' heels of human vulnerability to vibration. In addition, researchers have discovered an additional phenomenon of HAV known as "tonic vibration reflex" (TVR). At approximately 40 Hz, vibration seems to alter the muscle spindles and tendons of the hand elliciting a hand reflex. This reflex increases the grip force thus increasing the vibration coupling into the hand.[9]

SUMMARY

This introductory chapter describes the major principles involved in obtaining and analyzing vibration data impinging on the human hand. Topics briefly discussed include triaxial biodynamic and basicentric coordinate systems used for directly obtaining vibration measurements noninvasively from the human hand and methods for obtaining vibration measurements on vibrating hand tools respectively. A generic triaxial human vibration-measurement system is described, and methods of Fourier spectrum vibration data analysis and interpretation of an example spectrum are discussed. Engineering modeling of the human hand's response to vibration is discussed. The chapter concludes with an introduction to hand-arm resonances and TVRs and their relationship to vibrating hand tools commonly found in the work situation.

Notes
1. Wasserman, D. Human Aspects of Occupational Vibration. Amsterdam: Elsevier Publishers, 1987.
2. Wasserman, D.; Reynolds, D.; Behrens, V.; Taylor, W.; Samueloff, S.; Basel, R. "Vibration White Finger Disease in U.S. Workers Using Pneumatic Chipping & Grinding Hand-Tools." Vol. II *Engineering*. Cincinnati, Ohio: National Institute for Occupational Safety & Health, 1982; DHHS/NIOSH Publication No. 82-101.
3. Reynolds, D. "Hand-Arm Vibration: A Review of Three Years Research." In: Wasserman, D. and Taylor, W. eds. *Proceedings of the International Occupational Hand-Arm Vibration Conference*. Cincinnati: National Institute for Occupational Safety & Health, 1977: DHEW/NIOSH Publication No. 77-170.
4. Wasserman, *Human Aspects of Occupational Vibration*.
5. Coermann, R. "The Mechanical Impedance of the Human Body in Sitting and Standing Positions at Low Frequencies." *Human Factors* 1962; 4:225–230.

6. Wasserman, D. "Vibration:Principles, Measurements, and Health Standards." *Seminars in Perinatology* 1990; 14:311–321.
7. Wasserman, Reynolds, Behrens, Taylor, Samueloff, and Basel, "Vibration White Finger."
8. Reynolds, D.; Basel, R.; Wasserman, D.; Taylor, W. "A Study of Hand Vibration in Chipping & Grinding Operations: Power Levels Into the Hands of Operators of Pneumatic Tools Used in Chipping & Grinding Operations." *J. Sound & Vibration* 1984; 95:479–497.
9. Radwin, R.; Armstrong, T.; Chaffin, D. "Power Hand Tool Effects on Grip Exertions." *Ergonomics* 1987; 30:833–855.

10

Hand-Arm Vibration
Standards/Guides

D. E. Wasserman

The formulation of human-exposure standards for a given stressor represents the collection of much knowledge from laboratory and field research. These standards are modified periodically since our knowledge is constantly improving. A standard is based on the professional interpretation of the data available at that time. A consensus process. Because standards are issued at different times by different groups and countries using different data bases, assumptions, et cetera, they can vary somewhat from each other. This is true for vibration standards.

This chapter addresses the salient elements of hand-arm vibration (HAV) standards and guides used internationally, with emphasis on the United States and the United Kingdom. However, the reader is first cautioned not to attempt to use the information herein without first obtaining a complete copy of the specific standard or guide to be used and only after reading and understanding it completely.

Currently there are three human exposure to HAV standards/guides used in the United States, they are: ACGIH-TLV,[1] ANSI S3.34,[2] and the NIOSH HAV Criteria Document.[3] There is one U.K. standard, BS 6842[4] and one international standard ISO 5349.[5]

HISTORICAL PERSPECTIVE AND
INTERNATIONAL STANDARD ISO 5349.

The International Standards Organization (ISO), [Technical Committee 108, Subcommittee 4] first attempted to develop an HAV standard for human exposure in the 1960s. Russian, Japanese, and Czechoslovakian scientific deligations provided some of their initial laboratory response data and results.[6-8] These laboratory subjective response studies had to be used because of the paucity of HAVS epidemiology data. In these early studies, human subjects were asked to grasp handles that were attached to small vibrating shakers. Subjects were then asked to respond to the vibration intensity and frequency impinging on their hands as functions of exposure time. What emerged was a series of *weighted* "elbow shaped," time-dependent, daily vibration-dose curves similar to those shown in Figure 10-1.

These weighted curve shapes, together with some early vibrating-tool data, eventually became an integral part of the operative ISO HAV document known as ISO/DIS 5349, finally issued as ISO 5349 in 1986 after undergoing several revisions.[9] These daily ISO weighted vibration-dose curves themselves did not

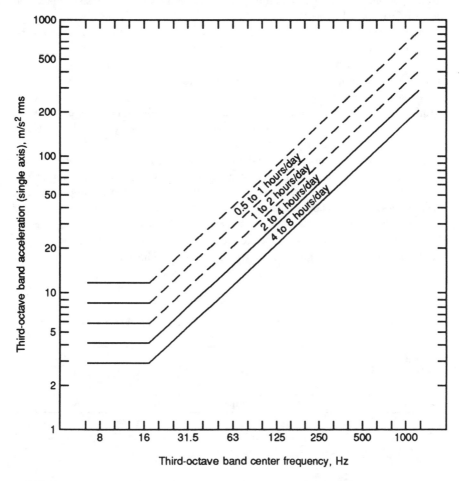

FIGURE 10-1.   Exposure zones as a function of daily hand-arm vibration exposure (ANSI S3.34-1986).

necessarily link yearly HAV exposure to the percentage of an exposed population who might experience the onset of HAVS symptoms. Brammer[10] subsequently reported the results of a review of many HAV studies. This data then became the basis of the current ISO 5349 dose-response section (see Figure 10-2), which was keyed to peripheral vascular stage 1, of the Taylor-Pelmear clinical assessment of HAVS developed in the United Kingdom.[11, 12]

In practice, to use ISO 5349, the daily weighted vibration exposure is determined for three perpendicular hand directions and then each result is separately normalized to a four-hour equivalent exposure for each axis (Figure 10-3). These results are then sequentially applied to a dose-response graph to determine the onset of HAVS peripheral vascular symptoms as a percentage of the exposed population (see Table 10-1 or Figure 10-2).

International Standards Organization 5349 provided what they believed to be the "weighted" shape (or envelope) of the human hand-arm response to HAV exposure (analogous to "A" weighting of the ear's response to sound). The ISO chose *not* to recommend acceptable human vibration intensity (acceleration) values for various exposure times throughout the workday. The ISO deferred to each country the choice of selecting their own acceptable weighted acceleration levels. As a result of this ISO action, virtually all HAV standards use this weighted measurement concept except for the NIOSH standard.

The critical issue at this time is whether the basic ISO human response curves are totally valid for the human hand-arm response to vibration from the plethora of vibrating tools used in the workplace. Some doubt exists on the application of these curves above 16 Hz because of the high-frequency vibration components of the newer faster tools.[13-16] This weighted curve shape is important since it determines how much of and at what frequencies the instrumentation records the vibration intensity impinging on the worker's hands. These measurement results

TABLE 10-1   Exposure Time in Years for Different Percentiles of a Population for Various Weighted Accelerations.

Weighted Acceleration (ah, w) eg (4)	Percentile of Population, C				
	10	20	30	40	50
m/sec./sec.	Exposure Time, Years				
2	15	23	>25	>25	>25
5	6	9	11	12	14
10	3	4	5	6	7
20	1	2	2	3	3
50	<1	<1	<1	1	1

Source: ISO 5349; 1986

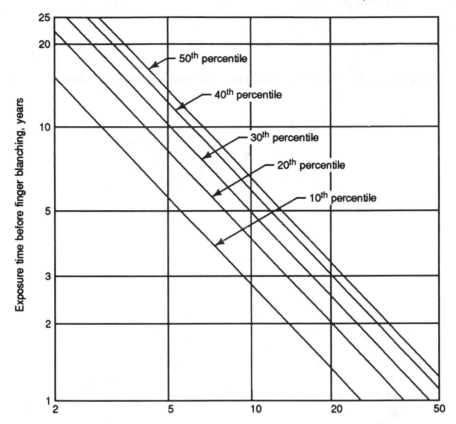

Values for r.m.s. weighted acceleration measured in a single-axis direction, m•s⁻²

FIGURE 10-2.   Exposure time for different percentiles of a population group exposed to vibration in three coordinate axes (ISO 5349-1986).

are then medically linked to weighted vibration levels. At present, HAV standards do not account for unweighted vibration levels.

GENERIC HAND-ARM VIBRATION STANDARDS FORMAT

Many HAV standards have a common *generic* series of necessary steps to be taken before using the standard, namely:

a. All HAV vibration measurements are obtained with reference to a uniform biodynamic and/or basicentric coordinate system. The former originates at

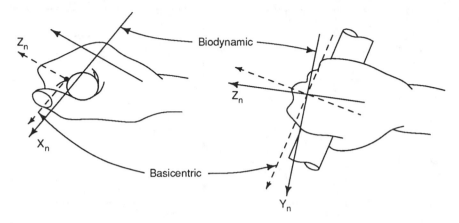

FIGURE 10-3.   Biodynamic and basicentric coordinate systems for the hand, showing the directions of the acceleration components for the assessment of hand-arm vibration (ACGIH-TLV, ANSI S3.34-1986, ISO 5349-1986).

the third metacarpal of the hand. The latter is obtained on the tool where the hand(s) grasp the tool (see Fig. 10-3).

b. Usually, the intensity measurement of choice is triaxial "root-mean-square" (rms) acceleration measurement, simultaneously obtained in the three perpendicular axes. Three independent accelerometers are used at each measurement point, averaged over a minimum of one minute continuous measurement time.

c. Both weighted and unweighted data should be obtained for each measurement axis.[17-21]

d. Data analysis is performed for each axis independently and includes a Fourier spectrum analysis, and/or values of both the overall weighted and unweighted (rms) acceleration for each axis.

e. Knowledge of the worker's daily exposure time is needed (for example, whether it is continuous or intermittent and/or different vibrating tools are used during the work shift).

f. Weighted data are also normalized in some standards to a four hour/day equivalent exposure. In the case of intermittent and/or different tool use during the work shift, a so-called "time weighted exposure average" must also be calculated.

g. An HAVS medical stage assessment using the Stockholm revised Taylor-Pelmear system,[22] is performed separately for each hand for both neurological and peripheral vascular symptoms.

h. The individual standard is next consulted to determine the resulting dose-response relationship.

Since calculations and procedures can and do vary among standards, obtain and carefully follow all the steps given in the standard you are using.

AMERICAN CONFERENCE OF GOV'T INDUSTRIAL HYGIENISTS: TLV

The ACGIH is a nongovernmental organization that in 1984 issued the first HAV standard in the United States[23] known as "threshold limit values" (TLV) as given in Table 10-2. In general, triaxial weighted vibration measurements are simultaneously obtained. The weighted acceleration values for each axis are next compared to Table 10-2 using the appropriate daily exposure times. If the (rms) acceleration levels of one or more axes are exceeded, then this standard has been exceeded. Caution must be exercised when evaluating higher frequency tools that may appear to fall within the standard. Both weighted and unweighted values as well as stage assessment should be noted. This standard covers vibration frequencies from 5.6–1,400 Hz. Recommended levels are keyed to not proceeding beyond a stage 1 medical assessment.

AMERICAN NATIONAL STANDARDS INSTITUTE: (ANSI) S3.34

American National Standards Institute S3.34 HAV standard was issued in 1986 and is shown in Figure 10-1. These are similar to the ISO-developed weighted curve

TABLE 10-2   Threshold Limit Values for Exposure of the Hand to Vibration in Either Xh, Yh, Zh Directions.

Total Daily Exposure Duration*	Values of the Dominant,† Frequency-Weighted, rms, Component Acceleration Which Shall Not be Exceeded** a_K' (aKeg)	
	m/s^2	g
4 hours and less than 8	4	0.40
2 hours and less than 4	6	0.61
1 hour and less than 2	8	0.81
less than 1 hour	12	1.22

*The total time vibration enters the hand per day; whether continuously or intermittently.
†Usually one axis of vibration is dominant over the remaining two axis. If one or more vibration axis exceeds the total daily exposure then TLV has been exceeded.
**1 g = 9.81 m/s ^{2}
Source: ACGIH.

shapes. The daily acceptable acceleration levels in Figure 10-1 have been chosen by ANSI. In practice, when using S3.34, this *same* graph is used to evaluate *each* vibration axis separately. The horizontal axis of Figure 10-1 shows vibration frequency in so-called 1/3 octave frequency bands extending from 5.6–1,400 Hz. The vertical axis shows vibration intensity in (rms) acceleration units of m/sec./sec., noting that 1g = 9.81 m/sec./sec. Each weighted curve is exposure-time dependent. To use ANSI S3.34, a Fourier spectrum analysis for each measurement axis is required, followed by a comparison of each vibration axis to the appropriate continuous daily exposure curve in Figure 10-1. This standard is exceeded if, one or more axes, the Fourier spectral peaks touch and/or pierce the selected daily exposure curve. Once the overall "weighted" (rms) acceleration values are obtained for each measurement axis, then each value must be compared or "normalized" to a four hour/day energy exposure. Finally, the resulting values are each sequentially applied (horizontal axis) to the graph shown in Figure 10-2, which shows the latent interval for a predicted percentage of the exposed population who most likely will begin the blanching process for a four hour/day normalized exposure. The latent interval is defined as the time it takes a worker to experience a first white fingertip from when he or she began using vibrating tools; this is shown in years in Figure 10-2 vertical axis.

In summary, ANSI S3.34 requires weighted vibration measurements and a spectrum analysis in three perpendicular axes; for each axis a determination is then made to see if the standard has been exceeded for various exposure times (Figure 10-2). The overall weighted measurement is compared to a four hour/day exposure in each axis. These results are used to predict the amount of time or latent interval a percentage of the total exposed population will begin the HAVS blanching process.

NATIONAL INSTITUTE FOR OCCUPATIONAL SAFETY AND HEALTH (NIOSH)

The NIOSH is a U.S. government agency established under the Occupational Safety and Health Act of 1971 as a research group with no regulatory powers, unlike its sister organization the Occupational Safety and Health Agency (OSHA). However, traditionally there has been a close working relationship between both agencies. The NIOSH, in 1989, was the third and last organization to publish a HAVS "criteria document" (#89-106) in the United States. In preparing this document, the NIOSH voiced concern over the shape of the weighted curves and their sufficiency to protect workers principally exposed to high-speed tools. Thus the NIOSH chose *temporarily not to issue any recommended exposure level* (REL) until new epidemiological studies become available, some of which have already begun to appear.[24-27] Recognizing the need for such standard, "NIOSH has therefore recommended a standard for exposure to HAV that includes no specific exposure limit but does include engineering controls, good work practices, use of protective clothing and equipment, worker training programs, administrative controls such as limited daily use time, and medical monitoring and surveillance." A cornerstone of the NIOSH standard is the requirement for medical monitoring of all vibration-exposed workers in order to identify the signs and symptoms of HAVS and to remove (at the stage 2 level) such workers from vibration exposure until they are free of all vibration-related symptoms.[28] The NIOSH document endorses previously discussed methods of vibration-dose measurement, analysis, and medical assessment for HAVS. The NIOSH document also requires:[29, 30] (a) weighted and unweighted triaxial acceleration measurements; (b) an extended frequency bandwidth from 5.6Hz to a new high-frequency limit of 5,000 Hz, not the 1,400 Hz in existing standards, thus encompassing the high-speed tool spectra, and (c) labeling of vibrating tools with their overall acceleration levels.

BRITISH STANDARDS INSTITUTION: (BSI) BS 6842

In the 1960s there began an intense effort by United Kingdom researchers to quantify the epidemiology and vibration spectral dose characteristics of gasoline-powered chain saws extensively used in United Kingdom forests.[31, 32] This action resulted in the BSI issuing, in 1975, a standard for development, standard DD 43 shown in Figure 10-4.

These are essentially ISO-type weighted curves for daily exposures of 150 and 400 minutes, the former established at 1 m/sec./sec., the latter at 10 m/sec./sec. In 1987 the BSI issued their revised document BS6842, which like ISO 5349, does *not* directly recommend specific acceptable HAV levels.[33] It does recommend using multiaxis weighted measurements and suggests that "it appears that, with normal tool usage, symptoms do not usually occur if the frequency weighted acceleration is below about 1 meter/sec./sec..." BS 6842 includes Table 10-3 showing the frequency weighted acceleration level values for 10 percent exposed populations expected to produce stage 1 finger blanching for daily exposures from 15 minutes to 8 hours. The dose-response graph does not appear in the document. Vibration dose is calculated on a normalized eight hour/day as opposed to a four hour/day as in ISO 5349. The frequency range is 8–1,000 Hz. Advice is also given on medical surveillance, measurements, and work practices.

SUMMARY

This chapter discusses the salient features and practical application of various HAV standards used internationally (ISO 5349), in the United Kingdom (BS

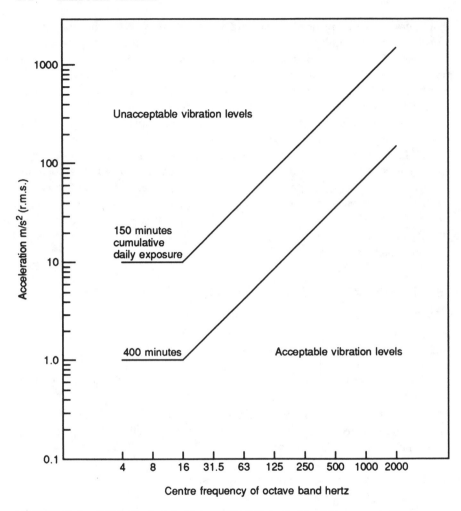

FIGURE 10-4.   British Standards Institute, DD43-1975 standard for the assessment of hand-arm vibration.

6842), and in the United States (ACGITH-TLV, ANSI S3.34, NIOSH Criteria Document). A brief historical perspective is given to clarify the genesis of these standards. Vibration measurements and data analysis are briefly reviewed for the reader in order to use and interpret these standards in a meaningful way. The issue of weighted versus unweighted measurements in these standards is discussed. In order to avoid potentially significant misapplication, the reader is advised to obtain and study a complete copy of the given standard before attempting to use it.

TABLE 10-3   Frequency Weighted Vibration Acceleration Magnitudes (m s -2 r.m.s.) Which may be Expected to Produce Finger Blanching in 10 percent of Persons Exposed. (BS6842:1987)

Daily Exposure	Lifetime Exposure					
	6 Months	1 Year	2 Years	4 Years	8 Years	16 Years
8 h	44.8	22.4	11.2	5.6	2.8	1.4
4 h	64.0	32.0	16.0	8.0	4.0	2.0
2 h	89.0	44.8	22.4	11.2	5.6	2.8
1 h	128.0	64.0	32.0	16.0	8.0	4.0
30 min	179.2	89.6	44.8	22.4	11.2	5.6
15 min	256.0	128.0	64.0	32.0	16.0	8.0

Note 1. With short-duration exposures the magnitudes are high and vascular disorders may not be the first adverse symptom to develop.

Note 2. The numbers in the table are calculated and the figures behind the decimal points do not imply an accuracy that can be obtained in actual measurements.

Note 3. Within the 10 percent of exposed persons who develop finger blanching, there may be a variation in the severity of symptoms.

Source: BS6842:1987.

Notes

1. American Conference of Goverment Industrial Hygienists. *Threshold Limit Values for Hand-Arm Vibration.* Cincinnati, OH 1990–91.
2. American National Standards Institute. S3.34. *Guide for the Measurement and Evaluation of Human Exposure to Vibration Transmitted to the Hand.* New York, N.Y. 1986.
3. National Institute for Occupational Safety & Health. *Criteria for a Recommended standard: Occupational Exposure to Hand-Arm Vibration.* 1989; DHHS/NIOSH Publication No. 89-106.
4. British Standards Institution. BS 6842 *Guide to the Measurement and Evaluation of Human Exposure to Vibration Transmitted to the Hand.* London, 1987.
5. International Standards Organization. ISO 5349. *Guidelines for the Measurement and Assessment of Human Exposure to Hand-Transmitted Vibration.* Geneva, 1986.
6. Wasserman, D. *Human Aspects of Occupational Vibration.* Amsterdam: Elsevier, 1987:188.
7. Miwa, T. "Evaluation methods for Vibration Effects-Measurements of Threshold and Equal Sensation Contours on the Hand for Vertical and Horizontal Sinusoidal Vibration." *Industrial Health* (Japan) 1967; 5:213–220.
8. Louda, L. "Mechanisms prevosu vibraci prumysloveko zdroje na cloveka." *CVUT Fakulta Stronjniho Inzenyrstvi.* Prague, 1965.
9. ISO 5399, *Guidelines.*
10. Brammer, A. "Threshold Limit for Hand-Arm Vibration Exposure Throughout the Workday." In: *Vibration Effects on the Hand and Arm in Industry.* New York: Wiley, 1982:291–301.
11. Taylor, W. (ed.) *The Vibration Syndrome.* London: Academic Press, 1987:226.

12. Taylor, W. and Pelmear, P., (eds.) *Vibration White Finger in Industry*. London: Academic Press, 1975:166.
13. Wasserman, D. "To Weight or Not to Weight....That is the Question." *J. Occup. Med.* 1989; 31:909.
14. Pelmear, P.; Leong, D.; Taylor, W.; Nagalingam, M.; Fung, D. "Measurement of Vibration of Hand-Held Tools: Weighted or Unweighted?" *J. Occup. Med.* 1989; 31:902-908.
15. Starck, J.; Pekkarinen, J.; Pyykkö, I. "Physical Characteristics of Vibration in Relation to Vibration-Induced White Finger." *Am. Ind. Hyg. Assoc. J.* 1990; 51:179-184.
16. Dandanell, R. and Engstrom, K. "Vibration From Riveting Tools in the Frequency Range 6 Hz-10MHz and Raynaud's Phenomenon." *Scand. J. Work. Environ. Health* 1986; 12:338-342.
17. NIOSH, "Criteria for a Recommended Standard."
18. Wasserman, "To Weight or Not to Weight."
19. Pelmear, Leong, Taylor, Nagalingum, and Fung, "Measurement of Vibration."
20. Starck, Pekkarinen, and Pyykkö, "Physical Characteristics of Vibration."
21. Dandanell and Engstrom, "Vibration From Riveting Tools."
22. Gemne, G.; Pyykkö, I.; Taylor, W.; Pelmear, P. "The Stockholm Workshop Scale for the Classification of Cold-Induced Raynaud's Phenomenon in the Hand-Arm Vibration Syndrome (Revision of the Taylor-Pelmear Scale)." *Scand. J. Work. Environ. Health* 1987; 13:275-278.
23. American Conference of Government Industrial Hygienists, *Threshold Limit Values*.
24. Wasserman, "To Weight or Not to Weight."
25. Pelmear, Leong, Taylor, Nagalingum, and Fung, "Measurement of Vibration."
26. Starck, Pekkarinen, and Pyykkö, "Physical Characteristics of Vibration."
27. Dandanell and Engstrom, "Vibration From Riveting Tools."
28. NIOSH, "Criteria for Recommended Standard."
29. Ibid.
30. Taylor, W. "Review: Occupational Exposure to HAV; the NIOSH Criteria Document." (U.K.) *Occup. Health Bull.* 1990; 3:4.
31. Taylor, *The Vibration Syndrome*.
32. Taylor and Pelmear, *Vibration White Finger*.
33. BS 6842, *Guide to the Measurement and Evaluation*.

11

The Control of Hand-Arm Vibration Exposure

D. E. Wasserman

The control of human exposure to hand-arm vibration (HAV) is usually multifaceted. The type and extent of the control measures depends largely on the severity and specifics of the given vibration hazard.[1, 2] The ergonomic and engineering approaches for controlling HAV are only part of the overall solution. Other additional controls include administrative action, personal protection, application of HAV standards, the use of antivibration tools, safe work practices, and finally medical monitoring of workers. These additional controls for HAV exposure are outlined elsewhere in this book.

The critical areas for HAV control are the vibrating tool source, the human receiver, and the pathway(s) between the source and receiver. The sources include worn bearings, unbalanced and excentric grinders and wheels, and unbalanced reciprocating forces. The hand–tool interface determines the vibration dose to the human receiver. Other factors influencing the receiver dose are the hand-arm system mass, spring and damping characteristics, resonances, and the hand's coupling/grip force characteristics.

Engineers mainly use two methods of reducing vibration: *isolation and damping*. Each method has its advantages and disadvantages, and in some instances both isolation and damping are used concurrently.

VIBRATION ISOLATION

Isolation is a method that alters or mismatches the pathway(s) between the vibrating source(s) and the human hand-arm receiver. If the mechanical coupling between the vibrating source and human receiver is reduced, and since coupling determines the overall amount of vibration transmitted to the hand-arm system, this results in less vibration impinging on the human (Figure 11-1).

175

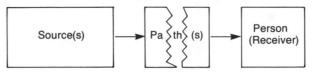

Isolation
Mismatch path(s) between source(s) & person
(receiver). Thereby gaining decoupling & a
lower transmissibility.

FIGURE 11-1.   Isolation is the mismatch path(s) between
sources(s) and person (receiver). Thereby gaining decoupling and
a lower transmissibility.

A graphic example of how the isolation principle operates is given in Figure
11-2. The goal is to redesign a cast aluminum automobile rocker cover, that was
causing excessive vibration to the vehicle. Vibration transmissibility is defined as
the ratio of output vibration to impinging input vibration as a function of vibration
frequency. The resultant ratio can take three forms. When the ratio equals one it
means that all the vibration going into a system emerges. When this ratio is less
than one it means that some of the incoming vibration is attenuated or reduced.
When the ratio is greater than one it means that what emerges is greater than the
input to the system, and we have a very undesirable condition known as "resonance." In Figure 11-2 the horizontal axis shows vibration frequency. On the
vertical axis is shown vibration transmissibility. The horizontal line given as ten
raised to the zero power (a number raised to the zero power is by definition equal
to one) is of interest because this is the unity line. The faulty rocker cover's vibration
response using a silicon gasket between it and the vehicle is shown as curve "A."
Its unwanted resonant peak appears at approximately 1,200 Hz. All of the area
under this "A" curve represents unwanted transmitted vibration. A specially designed nitrile rubber isolator gasket replaced the conventional silicon gasket and
the vibration test is repeated. The result is shown in curve "B." The resonant peak
has moved downward from 1,200 Hz to 120 Hz; a factor of ten in frequency
reduction *and* the transmitted vibration represented by all the area under the "B"
curve has also diminished. The resultant reduction of overall vibration transmission
is the difference in areas of graphs "A" and "B"; shown as "C" in Figure 11-2. This
is a significant reduction in vibration using isolation. An automobile shock absorber
is another example of an isolator, that minimizes, but does not totally eliminate,
road vibration.

VIBRATION DAMPING

Damping is a method of converting vibration energy into a small amount of heat.
This is accomplished by vibration forces impinging on and deforming viscoelastic

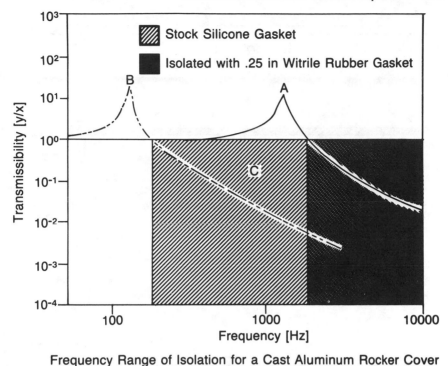

Frequency Range of Isolation for a Cast Aluminum Rocker Cover

FIGURE 11-2.   Frequency range of isolation for a cast aluminum rocker cover. Courtesy Anatrol Corp.

materials. The more efficiently the material converts mechanical vibration motion into heat, the better the damping material. These measures of efficiency are known as the material's "loss factor and storage modulus." [3,4] To determine these and other vibration characteristics, the material to be tested is applied to a bare steel beam approximately 12-inches long, 3/4-inch wide, 1/4-inch deep as in Figure 11-3. The material can be free layered either on the top and/or bottom along the beam length. Alternatively, the material can be "sandwiched" between two lengths of steel beam as in Figure 11-3-d. The steel/material laden beam is next placed in an environmental chamber and fixed at one end. The other end is free to move and bend up and down. Figure 11-4 shows the test setup. A magnetic vibrator is placed near, but not touching, the free end of the beam. Its purpose is to cause the beam to move and bend, up and down, in response to a computer-generated multiplicity of vibration signals, covering a large frequency spectrum called "white random noise" amplified by a power amplifier. At the fixed end of the beam is placed a piezoelectric vibration transducer, which senses this beam motion and converts it into a minute electrical signal, which is further amplified before going into a Fourier spectrum

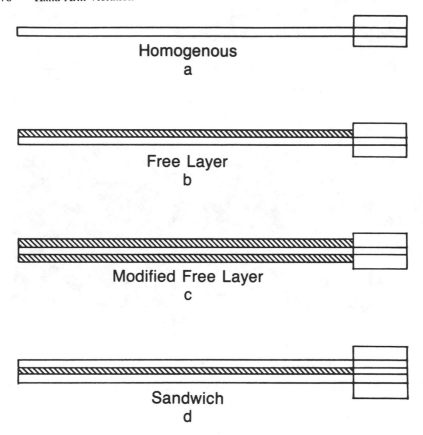

FIGURE 11-3.   Beam testing of materials.

analyzer. In the environmental chamber is a thermocouple, that monitors the temperature and transmits this information to a computer.

The purpose of this test is to determine the vibration-damping response characteristics of the material under test. The bare steel beam is used only as a support for the material. In the test, the beam is vibration excited over this broad frequency range as the chamber temperature is incrementally changed over a wide temperature range—from cold to warm to hot. The test is computer controlled, and covers a four-hour time period. The computer then automatically removes from the output data the "bare steel beam characteristics," leaving only the dynamic material properties (see Figure 11-5). The resulting three dimensional graphical computer output is called a "temperature spectrum map." Each material has a different map. A typical map is shown in Figure 11-6.

The horizontal axis of Figure 11-6 is vibration frequency, the vertical axis shows temperature, and the axis leaving the page is vibration intensity or amplitude. The

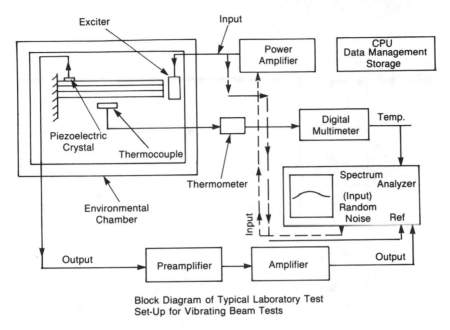

Block Diagram of Typical Laboratory Test
Set-Up for Vibrating Beam Tests

FIGURE 11-4.   Block diagram of typical laboratory test set-up for vibrating beam tests. Courtesy
Anatrol Corp.

traversed temperature range is subdivided into three regions: glassy (where the
material is stiff and cold); transition (where the material begins to warm); and
rubbery (where the material is pliable and hot). The material is never allowed to
liquify. There are a series of shifting "hills and valleys" coming out of the page.
These are the material's "resonances" and are called vibration modes. These resonances appear highest in amplitude in the glassy and rubbery regions. They are at
their lowest amplitude only in the transition region. The transition region is where
this material damps wideband vibration best because of the diminished hills and
valleys. The flatter and smoother the hills and valleys the better the damping material. If external vibration is applied to this material's glassy or rubbery region, and a
vibration frequency should coincide with a resonance peak of the material, *amplification* results, and the situation gets worse. The obvious conclusion is that in order to
be an effective damper of vibration a material must be used only in its transition
region and must be *matched or tuned* in its damping characteristics to that of the
vibration hand-tool source. To ignore material characteristics of matching or tuning
is to invite potential trouble because the material can be detrimental and actually
exacerbate the vibration impinging on the human. Since each material has its own
distinctive temperature map, and similarly each family of vibrating tools have their
own vibration spectra, it is highly unlikely that a single material can adequately

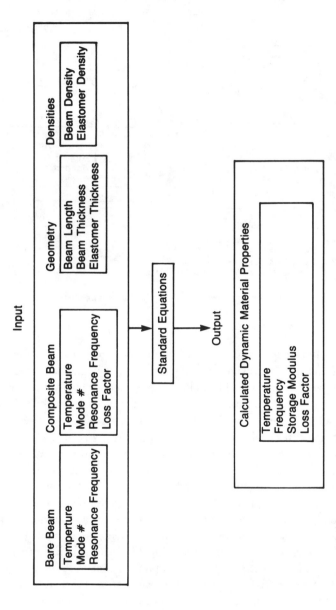

Data Reduction Process for the Calculation of Dynamic Material Properties Using the Vibrating Beam Technique

FIGURE 11-5. Data reduction process for the calculation of dynamic material properties using the vibrating beam technique.

Vibration Modes

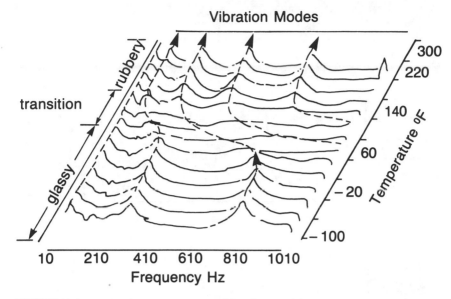

FIGURE 11-6.   A temperature spectrum map of damping material. Courtesy Anatrol Corp.

damp vibration from a variety of differing hand-tool sources. However, various materials, each with different characteristics, can be bonded together to produce the desired damping, where the use of a single material is not adequate. The effectiveness of a properly designed "damping treatment" is illustrated in Figure 11-7 and shows a "bare" untreated structure with its corresponding vibration spectrum. As matched damping material is applied to this structure the spectral peaks begin to diminish, and eventually most are removed. Applying material beyond a certain critical point cannot remove the remaining peaks.

Thus properly applied, vibration isolation and damping can be effective in minimizing harmful vibration from vibrating tools and along pathways. This principle also applies to antivibration protective gloves.

CONTROLLING HAND-ARM VIBRATION
USING ERGONOMIC AND OTHER METHODS

Ergonomics is the study of the interaction between the worker and the work process. When applying these principles to vibrating hand tools, the following points should be noted:[5]

a. A properly designed handle places minimum strain on the operator's hand and arm while keeping the wrist straight.
b. Tools should be designed for a high power-to-weight ratio.

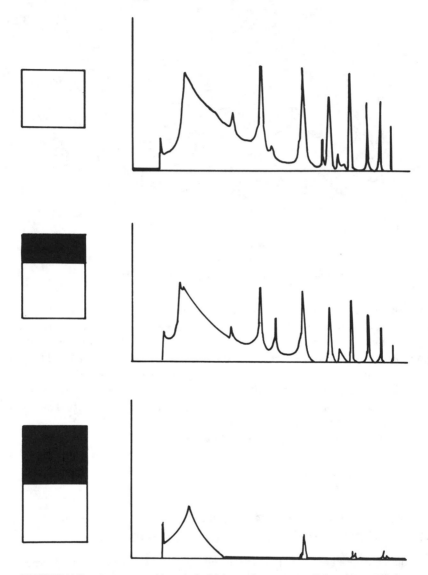

FIGURE 11-7. A structure without and with increasing amounts off damping material on the left, with corresponding spectra on the right. The vertical axis of the spectral graphs is amplitude, and the horizontal axis is vibration frequency. The spectra indicate significant effect of damping.

c. Various types of tool-handle configurations are optimized for specific jobs. These include "bow handles" used in chipping and large rivet hammers where the object is to transmit high feed forces with minimum wrist torque (Figure 11-8a). This occurs at an approximate natural angle of 70 degrees, the center line of the arm and wrist, as the tool is gripped. The "pistol handle" is used for precision tasks by keeping the tool length short and minimizing the bending forces on the wrists by keeping the tool's center of mass on top of the handle (Figure 8-b). Using a 70 degree natural angle, low grip forces transmit twist forces to the hand comfortably, whereas high grip forces keep the arm and wrist straight while transmitting high tool-feed forces to the work piece. Straight handles (Figure 11-8-c) are used for screwdrivers, drills, grinders, and nut runners. A diameter of 38 mm for men and 34 mm for women has been found to allow the strongest grip strength at minimum strain on the hand. For ease of movement, and precision work, at minimum wrist loading, the tool center of mass should be located where the tool is held with the distance kept short between work piece and hand. Using suspended tools

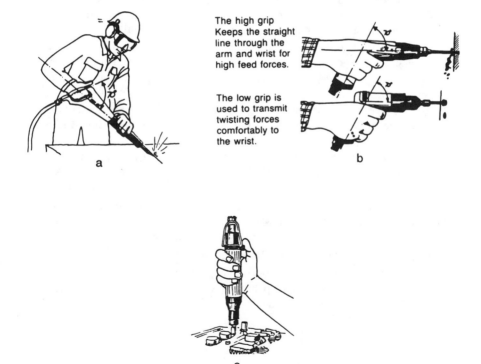

The high grip Keeps the straight line through the arm and wrist for high feed forces.

The low grip is used to transmit twisting forces comfortably to the wrist.

a

b

c

FIGURE 11-8.   Tool handle configurations. (a) Bow handle, (b) Pistol handle (c) Straight handle. Courtesy Atlas Copco Corp.

from the ceiling or mechanical arm "balancers" is desirable to minimize the tool weight and load on the worker.

d. Using worn-out tools, chucks, chisels, unbalanced grinding wheels, et cetera is undesirable since they usually exacerbate vibration tool levels.

e. Rerouting air exhaust tool lines away from the fingers and hands is desirable to minimize cold air exposure, which may induce blanching of fingers.

f. Workers are advised to let the tool do the work, gripping it as lightly as possible and safely, thereby minimizing the coupling of vibration into the hand.

g. Workers should use ergonomically designed "antivibration (A/V) tools" wherever and whenever possible to reduce vibration source levels. Antivibration chain saws and brush trimmers are readily available from numerous manufacturers. Currently, few A/V pneumatic tools are available. Some firms are placing warning labels on their tools and in the instruction books, while other firms are introducing ergonomically designed A/V pneumatic tools.

h. Since there are numerous conventional pneumatic tools currently in use, some users have attempted to reduce tool vibration levels by using inexpensive externally applied do-it-yourself tool sleeves. These should only be used as a *temporary measure*.[6] Properly designed A/V tools use specially designed isolators and/or damping treatments custom designed to optimize vibration attenuation characteristics, operating temperature range, and mechanical geometry. Experience has shown that no single damping or isolator material is satisfactory for a wide variety of tool types with different vibration spectral characteristics.

i. Use A/V gloves when and where possible. Optimally, A/V gloves should not only reduce vibration impinging on the hands of workers, but should also keep the hands warm, dry, and free of cuts and lacerations. Most critical is a proper glove fit and the ability of the glove to provide tactile feedback to the fingers, while still protecting the hands and fingers from harmful vibration. Proper tactile feedback ensures that the worker can safely grasp the hand tool with minimum grip force, and thus minimize vibration into the hands. Excessive grip force results in more vibration transmission to the hands, and will effectively mechanically "short circuit" the glove material's ability to adequately damp vibration. Finally, some manufacturers have chosen to solve the tactility problem by simply removing all finger protection, thus exposing the fingers leaving only palm and wrist protection. A "less than full finger glove" is NOT recommended.[7]

SUMMARY

This chapter discusses the engineering aspects of vibration and applied ergonomics to control HAV exposure. Topics include the principles and applications of vibration isolation and damping methods as applied to ergonomically designed tool and gloves. Ergonomic tool design, and a work practices guide to minimize vibration exposure to the hand and arm, are discussed.

Notes
1. Wasserman, D. *Human Aspects of Occupational Vibration*. Amsterdam: Elsevier, 1987; 188.
2. Wasserman, D. "The Control Aspects of Occupational Hand-Arm Vibration." *Applied Indust Hyg*. 1989; 4:F22–26.
3. Nashif, A. "Control of Noise and Vibration With Damping Materials." *Sound and Vibration* 1983; 17:28–36.
4. Nashif, A.; Jones, D.; Henderson, J. *Vibration Damping*. New York: Wiley, 1985.
5. Lindquist, B. "How to Design Vibration Controlled Power Tools." In: Lindquist, B, ed. *Ergonomic Tools in Our Time*.-Atlas Copco. Stockholm: TR Tryck, 1986:67–89.
6. Wasserman, "Control Aspects of Occupational Hand-Arm Vibration."
7. Ibid.

12

Hand-Arm Vibration Syndrome Legal and Compensation Aspects

D. Neusner (United States),
C. L. Arkell (United Kingdom)

As with all occupational illnesses there have been problems in recognizing and compensating workers with hand-arm vibration syndrome (HAVS). In Chapter 7 it will be noted how countries have differed in time when they first recognized HAVS. It is not surprising that legal and compensation practices have also varied. To enumerate the practices in all countries would be too wide ranging, so this chapter concentrates merely on two countries: the United States and the United Kingdom. It is, however, interesting to note that the Japanese litigation experience has been expensive and protracted, resulting in claimants failing to establish liability on their employers, with the courts taking the view, on the evidence, that HAVS was not a very serious disease.[1]

LEGAL ISSUES—UNITED STATES

At an oral presentation given in 1981 to fellow employees at the ARO Corporation, R. Stanley Short predicted "there will be growing liability arising from "hand-arm trauma" and that the 1980s would be[11] the decade of vibration." Stan Short was prophetic.

It has been an article of faith among many of the community interested in HAVS that it was difficult for HAVS patients in the United States to obtain compensation for their injuries.[2] Perhaps a more accurate statement would be that few workers with symptoms of HAVS were fairly compensated. This almost certainly resulted from a lack of understanding of the nature of HAVS among workers and many medical specialists. In giving occupational histories, workers commonly associated pain, numbness, tingling, or cold sensitivity in the hands with age, cold exposure, or nonspecific repetitive trauma. For their part, doctors tended to treat the symp-

186

toms of HAVS without regard to the cause, or make an incorrect diagnosis of carpal tunnel syndrome (CTS). An oft-seen phenomenon was the vibration-exposed injured worker who was diagnosed with CTS, treated surgically, and sent back to work with vibrating tools. Most of these workers would obtain little relief from surgery and go on to develop far more severe hand and arm symptomatology. Thus, while the high risk of injury was well documented in the literature, many vibration-exposed workers received inappropriate diagnosis and treatment and, as a consequence, insufficient compensation.

In the 1980s came a proliferation of workers' compensation and product liability claims for HAVS. There is nothing mysterious about this phenomenon—it was the inevitable consequence of workers, management, and the medical community becoming aware of the symptoms and causes of HAVS. In similar fashion, claims were first brought for asbestos disease in the early 1970s and for noise-induced hearing loss in the late 1970s. It was only with the acquisition of knowledge regarding the cause of their injuries that shipyard and factory workers came to understand that bad lungs and hearing loss were not inevitable consequences of age.

Another common thread linking these occupational diseases is the fact that manufacturers of the offending products were well aware of the risk of injury for many years before users. Juries have repeatedly found that asbestos manufacturers were aware of the risks of lung cancer and asbestosis prior to World War II.

Manufacturers of industrial machinery, including pneumatic tools, were aware of the association between noise exposure and hearing loss long before the U.S. Environmental Protection Agency (EPA) set safety standards for noise exposure.

Pneumatic tool manufacturers were made aware of the risks of vibration in 1918, when the U.S. Public Health Service published its study of stonecutting workers in Indiana.[3] Subsequent foreign studies of users of piston and rotary-operated vibrating tools drew attention to a high incidence of injury to the hands and arms. In 1947, Dart documented symptoms of HAVS among users of grinding and burring machines in the American aircraft industry.[4] Therefore, the risk of injury to vibration-exposed workers was well known over 50 years ago. Yet it is only within the last few years that tools manufacturers have begun to warn users of the known risk of vibration exposure.

In 1978, Black and Decker placed the following language in the safety instructions for its right-angle grinders:

> Continuous use of vibrating tools or use of vibrating tools by susceptible users may cause damage to hands.[5]

The other American manufacturers of pneumatic tools failed to use vibration warnings until 1987, when the Engineering Committee of the Compressed Air and Gas Institute voted to recommend that its members use the following warning on pneumatic tools:

Exposure to vibration may be harmful to your hands.

Many American manufacturers now place a decal with this or similar language on their hand-held pneumatic tools. These warnings may not provide sufficient information to allow users to make well-informed choices regarding tool use; nonetheless, the use of any vibration warning is certainly a welcome step toward the goal of designing safer tools and reducing injuries.

In response to the failure of manufacturers to warn of the risk of injury or take reasonable measures to make safer tools, hundreds of product liability lawsuits were brought against pneumatic tool manufacturers in the 1980s. At least one case, *Pultro v. Halite, Inc.* (filed in Middlesex County Superior Court, New Jersey) resulted in a plaintiff's verdict. Pultro involved a case of bilateral CTS resulting from long-term use of a pneumatic nail-gun. The plaintiff's testimony was that he used the tool an average of 150 times a day over a period of years. The plaintiff presented evidence that the tool did not have a warning regarding the risk of injuries to the hand and arm and, further, that the manufacturer had not taken technologically feasible steps to reduce vibration. An interesting aspect to this case was that the defendant did not dispute that vibration exposure was a competent producing cause of CTS.

Hundreds of lawsuits, yet to be decided, have been filed against manufacturers of chipping and grinding tools by workers at shipyards on the east coast. These cases are based on various theories of liability, including failure to warn and failure to utilize available antivibration technology. These plaintiffs also claim that the pneumatic tool industry collectively discouraged and inhibited development of warnings and safety standards. The plaintiffs used an assortment of chipping and grinding tools made by different manufacturers. Their injuries include vibration white finger (VWF); median and ulnar nerve disorders; and osteoarthritis of the hands, elbows, and shoulders.

While the outcome of the product liability litigation involving pneumatic tool manufacturers has yet to be decided, it is clear that the financial risk of litigation has had a salutory effect on actions of manufacturers, including the placing of warnings on many tools. Furthermore, there has been a significant increase in the number of tools incorporating antivibration designs. Most notably, Atlas Copco, a Swedish corporation, has introduced a complete line of vibration-reduced tools. Other U.S. manufacturers report that various antivibration designs for grinders are being developed.

A further incentive to the manufacturer of safer tools is the cost of workers' compensation claims to industrial users. Under the workers' compensation laws of the states and federal jurisdiction, employees are responsible for work-related injuries without regard to fault. Work injuries are characterized by their cause as either traumatic, repetitive trauma, or occupational disease. Hand-Arm Vibration Syndrome gives rise to a "repetitive trauma" or "occupational disease" claim, in the sense that it arises from a risk peculiar to the circumstances of employment. For most purposes, the semantic distinction among injuries is of little significance. To prove an injury compensable, a worker need only show that the circumstances of employment caused, contributed to, or aggravated a condition.

Vibration-exposed workers in the United States have complained of hand-arm symptoms for years. However, it is only within the last decade that compensation claims have been filed by large numbers of workers. It is the writer's experience, having handled over 300 claims for HAVS, that most factories and shipyards will accept such claims as readily as claims for traumatic injuries. What is usually required is a careful examination and testing of the patient, by a physician with relevant expertise, to make the correct differential diagnosis. Even in the presence of confounding conditions, such as diabetic neuropathy, rheumatoid arthritis, and sclerodema, the physician must consider whether vibratory exposure may have contributed to the overall impairment. A finding that vibration exposure was a contributing causative factor is sufficient to render the entire condition compensable.

When determining the degree of impairment due to HAVS, physicians and adjudicators of compensation claims often refer to the American Medical Association *Guides to the Evaluation of Permanent Impairment* (the "*Guides*"). The Third Edition of the *Guides* provides rating schemes for neurological and vascular disorders of the hands and arms in the "upper extremities" section. The *Guides* provide that assessments of impairment of the upper extremity be made based on pain, discomfort, sensory deficit, loss of strength, and cold sensitivity.[6]

In retrospect, it appears that the 1980s marked a crucial turning point in the struggle to obtain fair compensation for workers injured from vibration exposure. Hand-Arm Vibration Syndrome became firmly established in the United States as a recognized occupational disorder, as occupational physicians and hand specialists developed sophisticated diagnostic tools for making the differential diagnosis. Workers' compensation claims arising from vibrating tool use are now routinely accepted by factory and shipyard employers. Numerous product liability claims were filed against pneumatic tool manufacturers, which may result in additional relief to injured workers—but will certainly bring corollary benefits in the form of warnings and designs for safer tools.

COMPENSATION—UNITED KINGDOM

The compensation system in the United Kingdom has not yet caught up with HAVS. We are still talking in terms of VWF claims. Although the most recently decided common law claim to come before the court, *Smith and Loonat v. British Jeffrey Diamond Division of Dresser Europe S.A.*, was heard in June 1991, it related to matters dating back to 1982.

In the United Kingdom, there are three sources of compensation for the sufferer of VWF/HAVS: the state benefit scheme, a claim for damages at common law, and payment under an agreement between certain unions and certain employers' insurers.

State Benefit

Under the state industrial benefit scheme, a person who suffers injury or contracts a disease during the course of his or her employment may, if certain conditions are satisfied, be able to claim various benefits from the state for which he or she has paid through the National Insurance contribution system.

The State has long recognized certain diseases under this system, but it took 35 years for the Government to accept that "Vibration White Finger, also known as Raynaud's Phenomenon" should become a prescribed disease.

This system of compensation for diseases works on the basis of a specific definition for the disease with a further requirement for the sufferer to have been involved in one of a number of specific types of occupation.

In the case of VWF, the disease is defined as follows:[7]

"Episodic blanching, occurring throughout the year, affecting the middle or proximal phalanges, or in the case of a thumb the proximal phalanx, of:

a. in the case of a person with five fingers (including thumb) on one hand, any three of those fingers or
b. in the case of person with only four such fingers, any two of those fingers, or
c. in the case of a person with less than four such fingers, any one of those fingers or, as the case may be, the one remaining finger.

The types of occupation in which a person must have worked to be entitled to claim benefit for this condition are set out as follows:

a. the use of hand-held chain saws in forestry; or
b. the use of hand-held rotary tools in grinding or in the sanding or polishing of metal, or the holding of material being ground, or metal being sanded or polished, by rotary tools; or
c. the use of hand-held percussive metal-working tools, or the holding of metal being worked upon by percussive tools in riveting, caulking, chipping, hammering, fettling or swaging; or
d. the use of hand-held powered percussive hammers in mining, quarrying, demolition, or on roads or footpaths, including road construction; or
e. the holding of material being worked upon by pounding machines in shoe manufacturer."

It will be apparent from this description of the condition that it relates only to circulatory disturbance and has no reference to neurological symptoms.

Employees make their claims to their local Department of Health and Social Security Office (DHSS) by way of a standard claim form. The DHSS then has to decide a number of statutory questions to determine whether the employee qualifies for a payment of benefit. Claimants have to show that they had the appropriate employed earner's employment—any employment before 5th July 1948 does not qualify for benefit under the scheme. The DHSS has to be satisfied that the employee worked in a particular occupation for which the disease is prescribed.

There then has to be a diagnosis as to whether the claimant has the disease as defined in the Regulations, and that decision is made by an adjudication officer of the DHSS based on a medical report from a consultant, and advice from a regional medical officer of the DHSS. If the adjudicating officer is of the view that the claimant is suffering from the disease as prescribed, then the papers are referred to a Medical Board to consider the diagnosis and the extent of disablement. The Medical Board will examine the claimant and make its own assessment of the extent of the claimant's disability.

Experience has shown that many claimants under the scheme fail to satisfy the diagnostic criteria laid down by the Regulations.

Further, most cases of VWF that do meet those criteria are assessed at between 0 percent and 10 percent disablement. Since the Social Security Act of 1986, a minimum assessment of 14 percent is required for entitlement to disablement benefit for any condition, be it due to injury or disease, so that many claimants for VWF do not now receive benefits.

For those claimants who can overcome the diagnostic criteria relating to episodic blanching, the Medical Board will take into account in the assessment of disability any neurological problems that the claimant has as a result of his or her condition. This means that the DHSS scheme recognizes the neurological aspects of vibration syndrome, but as secondary to the vascular component.

It is unfortunate for someone who has had neurological symptoms from exposure to vibration but who does not have the requisite vascular symptoms. He or she would be outside the scope of the prescribed disease and would not be entitled to benefits.

With regard to the amount of benefits to which a successful claimant is entitled, this will depend on the percentage assessment above 14 percent. Past claimants whose income has been reduced as a result of the disease have been paid reduced earnings allowance in addition to disablement benefit, but reduced earnings allowance has now been discontinued as part of government policy to reduce all state benefits.

Claims For Damages at Common Law

The second way in which a person can seek compensation is by way of a claim for damages at common law through the civil courts.

There has been no coherent development in claims for compensation for VWF. This is because of the way in which the legal system works. In the United Kingdom, the adversarial nature of the legal system means that the result of a claim for damages depends entirely on the evidence presented to the judge. The judge is not in the position of an inquisitor and can only make decisions on the evidence before the court. It is therefore in the hands of the parties to an action exactly what evidence they present to the court.

This raises the question of the costs of litigation, since the quality of the evidence presented to the court can depend on how much a party is willing or able to spend on expert and medical evidence.

In the United Kingdom, the principle is that the losing party pays both parties' costs, therefore costs are an important consideration. (Proposals are currently being considered that could modify that principle to some degree for personal injury claims.)

In practice, the majority of common law claims for damages for VWF are brought by employees against their employers for exposure to vibration during the course of their employment. The writer knows of no claims for damages for VWF brought by a sufferer against the manufacturers of pneumatic or other vibration-producing tools.

Most plaintiff employees bring their claims backed by a trade union, which union will cover the costs involved in the claim on behalf of the employee. The claims are defended by the insurers of the plaintiff's employer.

Although these litigants have an advantage over litigants not backed by unions or insurers, or by the Legal Aid Fund of access to resources, contrary to popular belief, neither the trade unions nor the insurers have a bottomless pit of money to spend on litigation. This can circumscribe the technical and medical evidence presented to the court.

Claims for damages for VWF, like other personal injury claims, are brought in negligence, a tort, or civil wrong. The plaintiff must show the existence of a duty of care owed to him or her by the defendant. That duty is to take reasonable care to avoid causing injury or damage to the plaintiff. The plaintiff must then prove a breach of that duty to take reasonable care, which has resulted in damage or injury to him or her. If he or she can prove a breach of duty causing damage, then the tort of negligence is complete and he or she will be entitled to compensation.

The reason why there have been no claims for damages for VWF against manufacturers of vibration-producing tools is probably that sufferers from VWF have usually contracted their condition when using vibrating tools in the course of their employment. In the United Kingdom, the law has developed so that employers have a very high duty with regard to the safety of their employees. In addition to the employer's common law duty of care, Parliament has laid down extensive statutory duties on the employer for the safety of employees, which often impose strict liability. In this climate, the courts have tended to interpret quite strictly the employer's common law duties toward employees. In these circumstances, it is generally easier for an employee to prove that his or her employer was negligent or in breach of statutory duty than it would be for him or her to prove negligence on the part of the manufacturer of the vibration-producing tool.

The question of whether an employer is in breach of duty to take reasonable care for the safety of employees depends on what knowledge the employer has or ought to have concerning the potential injury involved in a certain situation or process, how serious the potential injury to the employee would be if any particular risk of injury should materialize, and the cost to the employer in terms of time and money in guarding against that risk.

The law does not require an employer to take expensive precautions to guard against a small risk of trivial injury, whereas it will require an employer to take such precautions to guard against a small risk of a serious injury. The question of the extent of the risk has also to be considered by the employer so that a serious risk of a trivial injury may warrant precautions.

There is therefore no general rule that can be laid down as to whether a particular claimant would succeed in any particular claim against an employer. It depends on the evidence that is presented to the court. Thus, although Mr. Justice Kilner-Brown in his judgment in *Heal v. Garringtons Limited* (26th May 1982; unreported, save in Kemp and Kemp "the Quantum of Damages" Volume 2 Para 9-854/1. Sweet and Maxwell.) indicated that he thought there was sufficient medical and scientific evidence to put employers as a whole on the alert as to VWF from 1976 onwards, that decision would not bind a judge in another case to hold that that was the date of knowledge, though in practice, some solicitors and insurers dealing with such claims take 1976 as the generally accepted date of knowledge. Date of knowledge does not always equate with date of liability, since once an employer is found to have had actual or constructive knowledge, he or she has to be given a chance to react to that knowledge before being found negligent.

In *Shepherd v. Firth Brown Limited*, decided by Mr. Justice McCullough in 1985 (17th April 1985; unreported), he considered that the defendant had actual knowledge of the problem of VWF in the Spring of 1976 but he allowed the defendants a notional three years in which to have done something about the problem so that he found that liability only attached from 1979.

The date of liability can be very important with regard to the assessment of the amount of compensation, since the cases show that most judges will make an apportionment of the amount of damages awarded on the basis of "guilty" years as a proportion of total years' exposure. Most plaintiffs have had many years' exposure to vibration before they institute a claim for damages. Take a man employed on vibration-exposed work since 1960 whose claim is determined in 1990. The court would first have to decide if the employer was negligent. Suppose the judge found negligence from 1976. The court would then assess the extent of the disability as at 1990, but would make some apportionment to take account of the fact that although the condition had been caused by exposure over 30 years, only 14 of those years related to the period when the employer was negligent.

How much the claimant would receive would depend to a large extent on whether there was any reliable evidence of the stage his condition had reached as at 1976 or whether he could indicate retrospectively the state of his condition at that time.

The amount of compensation actually awarded by judges, ignoring the question of apportionment, has varied widely. In cases in which evidence has been given stressing the triviality of the condition, the judges have treated the condition accordingly.

Mr. Justice Kilner-Brown in *Heal v. Garringtons Limited* did not accept that the condition was a trivial one and he based his assessment of damages on the Taylor-Pelmear scale.[8] He endeavoured to lay down a general tariff for VWF from inception to Stage 4, and the figures he put on the stages (having heard the detailed effects of the condition) were generally in line with the sorts of awards of damages being given for other personal injuries. In the *Heal* case, there was no emphasis on the sensory problems associated with VWF.

In the later series of cases, of *McFaul and Others v. Garringtons Limited* (9th November 1984; unreported), Mr. Justice Hodgson rejected the use of the Taylor-Pelmear scale as a method of assessing damages and took considerable note of the effects of the condition on an individual's activities, and he emphasized the loss of amenity aspect.

He valued the worst case of VWF in 1984 at a figure that equated the condition, in terms of disability, with someone who had had some of his fingers amputated in an accident and had a permanent loss of dexterity.

In the most recently reported case of *Smith and Loonat v. British Jeffrey Diamond Division of Dresser Europe S.A.* (19th June 1991; unreported), the judge, Mr. Justice Swinton Thomas, said of VWF:

"It must be appreciated that vibration white finger, although very unpleasant, is not dangerous to life or general health. In some respects it might perhaps be compared to a workman, doing heavy work, having a bad back. The condition escalates but then reaches a plateau."

He did not make an assessment of the amount of appropriate compensation because he found that the plaintiffs had failed to establish that their employers were negligent.

The Agreement

The third method of compensation for sufferers of VWF is under an agreement made between the General Municipal Boilermakers and Allied Trades Union

(GMBATU) and the Iron Trades Insurance Company in 1985. This agreement came about because both the union and the insurance company had been involved in a large amount of expensive litigation over many claims for VWF with erratic results.

To avoid the expense of litigating in claims relating to exposure to vibration, this agreement provided for the compensation of sufferers from VWF provided certain conditions were met. The schedule of compensation is based on a classification of the claimant's condition on the Taylor-Pelmear scale with payments of modest amounts for pain and suffering and loss of amenity. There is provision in the agreement for an additional payment to a claimant who can prove that he or she has sustained a loss of earnings, loss of promotion, or will sustain loss of earnings in the future by reason of his or her condition, that sum to be negotiable. If a claimant accepts a payment under the agreement, it is a condition that that sum is accepted in full and final settlement of any claim at common law.

Other unions and insurers have become signatories to the agreement, recognizing the benefits to both the union members and to employers' insurers in avoiding the uncertainties of litigation over VWF claims.

The unions cannot bind their individual members to the agreement, but many people have taken advantage of the agreement and have been compensated quickly, avoiding lengthy and expensive litigation.

There are still a number of cases that are pursued at common law outside the agreement, but these cases have been settled by negotiation between the parties to avoid the additional costs and uncertainty of proceeding to trial.

Avoiding Litigation

Common law claims for damages for VWF involve the plaintiff employee proving fault on the part of the defendant employer. It has been accepted by judges in VWF claims that the test to be applied in deciding whether an employer has been negligent is the test propounded by Mr. Justice Swanwick in *Stokes v. G.K.N. (Nuts and Bolts) Limited* (1968; 1 W.L.R. 1776), in which he stated:

"The overall test is still the conduct of the reasonable and prudent employer, taking positive thought for the safety of his workers in the light of what he knows or ought to know; where there is a recognised and general practice which has been followed for a substantial period in similar circumstances without mishap, he is entitled to follow it, unless in the light of commonsense or newer knowledge, it is clearly bad; but where there is developing knowledge, he must keep reasonably abreast of it and not be too slow to apply it; and where he has in fact greater than average knowledge of the risks, he may thereby be obliged to take more than the average or standard precautions. He must weigh up the risk in terms of the likelihood of injury occurring and the potential consequences if it does; and he must balance this against the probable effectiveness of the precautions that can be taken to meet it and the expense and inconvenience they involve. If he is found to have fallen below the standard to be properly expected of a reasonable and prudent employer in these respects, he is negligent."

This proposition was adopted and extended by Mr. Justice Mustill in *Thompson v. Smiths Ship Repairers Limited* (1984; 1 A11 E.R. 881), in which he cited the previously cited proposition of law and went on to say as follows:

"Swanwick J. drew a distinction between a recognised practice followed without mishap and one which in the light of common sense or increased knowledge is clearly bad. The distinction is indeed valid and sufficient for many cases. The two categories are not, however, exhaustive, as the present actions demonstrate. The practice of leaving employees unprotected against excessive noise had never been followed 'without mishap.' Yet even the Plaintiffs have not suggested that it was 'clearly bad,' in the sense of creating a potential liability in negligence, at any time before the mid-1930s. Between the two extremes is a type of risk which is regarded at any given time (although not necessarily later) as an inescapable feature of the industry. The employer is not liable for the consequences of such risks, although subsequent changes in social awareness, or improvements in knowledge and technology, may transfer the risk into the category of those against which the employer can and should take care. It is unnecessary, and perhaps impossible, to give a comprehensive formula for identifying the line between the acceptable and the unacceptable. Nevertheless, the line does exist, and was clearly recognised in *Morris v. West Hartlepool Steam Navigation Company Limited* (1956 1. All E.R. 385). The speeches in that case show, not that one employer is exonerated simply by proving that other employers are just as negligent, but that the standard of what is negligent is influenced, although not decisively, by the practice in the industry as a whole. In my judgement this principle applies not only where the breach of duty is said to consist of a failure to take precautions known to be available as a means of combating a known danger, but also where the omission involves an absence of initiative in seeking out knowledge of facts which are not in themselves obvious. The employer must keep up to date, but the Court must be slow to blame him for not ploughing a lone furrow."

An employer must be shown to have some knowledge about the risk of HAVS before he or she can be said to be in breach of his or her duty of care to the employee to reduce that risk. Where an employer cannot be shown to have actual knowledge of the risk of HAVS, a judge may nevertheless conclude that in the light of general knowledge in the industry and knowledge disseminated in industrial and medical journals and the like, an employer should have known of the risk.

It appears that HAVS has been experienced by users of vibrating tools ever since such tools were brought into general use in industry. In the past, the condition has been accepted as part of the job in cases where the employees actually attributed the symptoms to the job and did not merely dismiss them as "one of those things." However, knowledge of the condition has increased and employees are now less prepared to tolerate inconvenience and pain that they might, in the past, have accepted.

Once an employer is fixed with knowledge, actual or constructive, of the risk of HAVS from processes within his or her factory, he or she must decide what steps to take in the light of that knowledge.

An employer should consider practical measures that might be taken to reduce vibration from processes within the factory. It may be possible to eliminate vibration from the work by changing the way in which the work is done, or automating the process. An employer should consider in particular, the tools in use in the factory, and whether these can be replaced with vibration-damped tools. Improved maintenance of tools might help reduce the vibration.

An employer should also consider whether he or she could reduce employees' exposure to vibration by reducing the amount of time they work with vibrating tools. In some factories and on certain processes, it might be possible to reduce exposure by the rotation of workers between vibration-exposed and non-vibration-exposed jobs. The practicability of this will depend on the skills required by the personnel in the factory, and many employers find that in practice, because employees working with vibration tools are generally paid a higher wage than those working on non-vibration-exposed jobs within the factory, it is impossible to implement an effective rotation system.

An employer should also try to keep up to date with practical developments with regard to the reduction of vibration, and to keep in contact with the health and safety executive and his or her own trade association with regard to such developments.

In some cases, an employer might have to take the advice of an outside specialist with regard to the means of protecting employees from excessive vibration. If such an expert is engaged to advise, then the employer must be very careful to follow up any advice given. If any part of the expert's advice is rejected, a record should be kept of the detailed reasons why the advice was not followed, for example, prohibitive cost. An employer who engages an expert and then fails to act on that expert's advice, would be in danger of being held negligent in any future litigation.

Expert advice may involve vibration measurement and comparison of the levels of vibration from various tools and processes with the recommended levels for safe working to be found in, for example, B.S.I. 6842.[9]

The employer should also take steps to improve the environment for employees. Attacks of VWF could be minimized by maintaining a reasonable temperature in the workplace, and by providing a restroom where employees can warm their hands if an attack does occur. Some of the steps suggested may not be practicable for a particular employer, but the law requires that such steps should be considered.

The employer should also keep a dated record of the practical steps he or she has considered and rejected, those steps he or she has considered and tried to develop, and those steps that have been successful. In any future litigation, he or she can then produce contemporaneous evidence of what has been done.

The most important single step an employer should take is to give advice and information to employees of the risk of HAVS. In the past, some employers have deliberately not instituted any warning system of the risks of HAVS to avoid stirring up "a hornet's nest." There was a fear that by warning employees, they would create needless alarm and, incidentally, but probably more importantly, they might provoke litigation.

An employer should provide information to employees concerning the risks and effects of the condition so that the employees are fully informed as to the risks they are running in their employment and the consequences. It is particularly important to give accurate advice in this respect and this is a particular area where it may be necessary to obtain outside assistance, for example from the Health and Safety Executive, or from the Employment Medical Advisory Service.

To protect the employer's position so far as any future litigation is concerned, he or she should keep a careful note of the information provided to employees. Employees should be individually warned and a record kept of the exact nature of the warning and the date it was given. This matter can be approached by drawing up a standardized leaflet setting out in layman's terms an explanation of HAVS and its causes, and its progressive nature. A verbal warning could then be given along the lines of the leaflet, and a copy of the leaflet handed to the employee to keep, with a record in the employee's personnel records that the warning and leaflet have been given on a particular date. It is important to have available someone who might be able to answer queries from the employees concerning the condition.

Warnings should run hand in hand with some procedure for regular checks on the employee's condition so that an individual employee's condition can be monitored and the employee kept informed with regard to the inception or progression of the disease. This is a matter best done by an employer's Medical Department or by someone medically qualified and with knowledge of HAVS. Again, detailed records of the examinations should be kept. Even today, there is a risk in leaving employees to the mercy of their general practitioners (GP) so far as advice on the disease is concerned, since many GPs still seem to have very little knowledge of the condition.

The question has arisen in the past as to whether an employer should force an employee off the job when a certain stage of the disease is reached. The type of risk involved with HAVS is not such that an employer is required to take such drastic action in the normal case, though there might be a greater risk for an individual employee who was unusually susceptible to the disease. Provided that an employer gives employees all relevant information concerning the disease and its progression, with appropriate medical advice, then it is reasonable to allow employees to decide whether to continue with vibrating work, because they can make informed decisions. This was the approach adopted by Mr. Justice Swinton Thomas in the case of *Smith and Loonat v. British Jeffrey Diamond Division of Dresser Europe S.A.*

It is also important for an employer to keep a record of employees who fail to cooperate with any system of medical checks or counseling.

All common law claims are decided by the judge on the evidence presented. An employer might take all the various precautions outlined, and still be found liable for failing to take reasonable care, because of the way in which the particular judge interprets the evidence. This is why the writer has elsewhere described the common law claims on VWF as "the Lottery of Litigation." [10]

The Future

In current claims for damages for HAVS, the medical evidence put forward has started to refer to more sophisticated methods of assessing the condition than the Taylor-Pelmear scale, and there are now references to the Stockholm scale[11] appearing in medical reports. In future cases, judges will undoubtedly be presented with more advanced evidence both from medical experts and from engineering experts, which will change the court's approach to claims based on exposure to vibration and will give recognition to HAVS. In practice, the more serious the condition of HAVS is shown to be by evidence before a court, the stricter will be the standards applied by the courts in judging an employer's actions.

SUMMARY

In this chapter the legal and compensation issues in respect of HAVS are reviewed for two countries only: the United States and the United Kingdom. It will be noted that in the United Kingdom the primary benefit to workers suffering from HAVS has been obtained through common law claims via the law courts. State benefit has been less effective, and as a result of recent legislation a minimum disability of 14 percent is required for entitlement. Consequently even fewer workers will benefit. In the United States, state benefit has been the primary vehicle, but litigation for product liability with tool manufacturers is now being pressed.

Notes
1. Welfare Division of Administrative Department, Forestry Agency of Japan. "A Summary of Hand-Arm Vibration Syndrome Judgements—*Matsumoto et al.* (of the Forestry Agency workers) *v. the State* (the Forestry Agency). 1991:28
2. Wasserman, D., ed. *Human Aspects of Occupational Vibration*. New York: Elsevier, 1987:188.
3. Hamilton, A. "A Study of Spastic Anasmia in the Hands of Stonecutters. Effect of the Air Hammer on the Hands of Stonecutters." U.S. Bureau Labor Stat. 1918; 19: Bulletin 236: 53–66.
4. Dart, E. E. "Effects of High Speed Vibrating Tools on Operators Engaged in the Airplane Industry." *Occup. Med.* 1946; 1:515–550.
5. "Black and Decker Owners' Manual for Right Angle Grinders, Safety Instructions." 1978 (July); Publication No. 17.

6. American Medical Association. *Guides to the Evaluation of Permanent Impairment.* 3rd ed. 1988;42–44.
7. The Social Security (Industrial Injuries) (Prescribed Diseases) Regulations 1985 S.I. 1985/967.
8. Taylor, W. and Pelmear, P. L., eds. *Vibration White Finger in Industry.* London: Academic Press, 1975:166.
9. British Standards Institution BS 6842. *Guide to Measurement and Evaluation of Human Exposure to Vibration Transmitted to the Hand.* London, HMSO, 1987.
10. Arkell, C. "The Lottery of Litigation." In: Aw, T. C., Cooke, R. A., Harrington, J. M., Krishnan, G., and Taylor, L. E., eds. Proceedings of a Symposium on the Assessment and Associated Problems of Vibration White Finger. Institute of Occupational Health, University of Birmingham, 1989:No.2;129.
11. Gemne, G., Pyykko, I., Taylor, W., and Pelmear, P. L. "The Stockholm Workshop Scale for the Classification of Cold-Induced Raynaud's Phenomenon in the Hand-Arm Vibration Syndrome (revision of the Taylor-Pelmear Scale)." *Scand. J. Work. Environ. Health* 1987; 13:275–278.

Appendix 1

Hand-Arm Vibration Syndrome

Health Surveillance Pre-Placement Initial Assessment

Date ___/___/____

SECTION 1   PERSONAL IDENTIFICATION

Last Name_____Date of Birth ___/___/____

First Name_____ Tel. No _____

Address _____

_____

Works/WCB No. _____ Department _____

Health/National Insurance Number____/____/____

Sex: M / F   Dominant hand: Left / Right

Family Physician's Name _____

Address _____

_____

Telephone Number (   ) _____

SECTION 2   VIBRATION EXPOSURE HISTORY

a. *Present Occupation*   Company _____

Job title _____

Description of work _____

Tools used _____

_____

Date started present job___/___/19 _____

Approximate time exposed to vibration:

Hours per week _____

Weeks per year _____

No. of years_____

b. *Past Occupations* (list others overleaf):

	1	2	3
Company	_____	_____	_____
From/to	_____	_____	_____
Job title	_____	_____	_____
Tools used	_____	_____	_____
	_____	_____	_____
	_____	_____	_____
	_____	_____	_____
Vibration Exposure hrs. per week	_____	_____	_____
Weeks per year	_____	_____	_____
No. of years	_____	_____	_____

	4	5	6
Company	_____	_____	_____
From/to	_____	_____	_____
Job title	_____	_____	_____
Tools used	_____	_____	_____
	_____	_____	_____
	_____	_____	_____
	_____	_____	_____
Vibration Exposure hrs. per week	____	____	____
Weeks per year	____	____	____
No. of years	____	____	____

SECTION 3   MEDICAL HISTORY

a. *Constitutional White Finger* (Raynaud's Disease)

   i. As a young person did your fingers go white in the cold?   Yes / No

   ii. How old were you when this began to happen_____(Age in years)

   iii. Does it still occur?   Yes / No

   iv. If so, which fingers are affected? Specify with distribution:

	RL	RR	RM	RI	RT	LT	LI	LM	LR	LL	Fin.Th.	Score
Dist.	__	__	__	__	__	__	__	__	__	__	1	4
Mid.	__	__	__	__			__	__	__	__	2	-
Prox.	__	__	__	__	__	__	__	__	__	__	3	5

Score Right_____   Score Left_____   Total_____

   v. Are your toes also affected?   Yes / No

   vi. How often does it occur?_____

vii. Does it affect anyone else in your family? Specify: Yes / No

_____

b. *Injury*

i. Have you ever injured your hands, arms, shoulders, or neck, including the blood vessels?   Yes / No

ii. If yes, (a) specify part affected, type of injury, fracture, etc.

_____ date _____

_____

(b) has it left any residual effects? If so specify:

_____

c. *Connective Tissue Disorders*

i. Have your suffered from a connective tissue (collagen) disease? exempli gratia, systemic lupus erythematosus, polyarteritis nodosa, scleroderma, rheumatoid arthritis, dermatomyositis, Dupuytren's contracture.   Yes / No

ii. If yes, (a) specify which, and when it began: _____

(b) are you still receiving treatment? If so, specify: _____

_____

(c) has the disease caused any lasting effects? _____

_____

Specify: _____

_____

d. *Vascular Disorders*

i. Do you suffer, or have you suffered from:

a. High blood pressure   Yes / No
b. Ischaemic heart disease (angina)   Yes / No
c. Intermittent claudication   Yes / No
d. Migraine   Yes / No
e. A clotting tendency, including thrombosis in hand or arm   Yes / No

ii. Are you still receiving treatment? If so specify: Yes / No

_____

iii. Has the disease caused any lasting effects? If so specify: Yes / No

_____

e. *Neurological Disorders*

    i. Have you ever suffered from any chronic neurological disorder? exempli gratia, polio, syringomyelia, stroke or multiple sclerosis. Yes / No

    ii. If yes, specify what disorder and when you were affected:_____

_____

    iii. What treatment did you receive?

_____

    iv. Has the disease caused any lasting effects?

_____

f. *Degenerative Diseases*

    i. Have you ever suffered from arthritis of, or disc lesions in the neck?   Yes / No

    ii. Have you ever suffered from soft tissue or joint disorders in the arm or hand?   Yes / No

    iii. Have you suffered from carpal tunnel syndrome?   Yes / No

    iv. If yes to any of the above, specify which and when you were affected:

_____

    v. Are you still receiving treatment? If so, specify:

_____

    vi. Has the disease caused any lasting effects? If so, specify:

_____

g. *Other Chronic Illness*

    i. Do you suffer from any chronic illness not specified above? exempli gratia, diabetes or thyroid disease.   Yes / No

    ii. If yes, specify:_____

_____

h. *Treatment*

    i. Are you taking any medication regularly?   Yes / No

    ii. If yes, specfy:_____

SECTION 4   SOCIAL HISTORY

a. *Smoking*

    i. Do you smoke, or have you ever smoked?   Yes / No

    ii. When did you start smoking regularly?   19____

    iii. (Ex-smokers) When did you stop smoking?   19____

    iv. How much do you/did you smoke?

                              cigarettes/cigars____   per day

                              pipe/rolling tobacco____oz per day

                              number pack years*____

b. *Alcohol*

    i. Do you or have you ever consumed alcohol?   Yes / No

    ii. Do you drink only socially?   Yes / No

    iii. (Ex-drinkers) When did you stop?   19____

    iv. If a regular drinker, how many units do you

           drink per day/week?   _____day/week

           1 unit = 1 bottle/pint beer, single spirit, glass wine.

c. *Hobbies/Leisure Pursuits*

    i. Do you have any hobbies?   Yes / No

      If yes, specify:_____

      _____ _____

    ii. Do you engage in outdoor pursuits or gardening?

      Specify: Yes / No

      _____

    iii. Specify any restriction:_____

    iv. Do you now, or have you in the past used any of the following
       tools regularly at home or away from work?

_____

*Number of cigarettes smoked a day × number of years smoked divided by 20 = number of pack years.

	Current user	Past user
Chain saw	Yes / No	Yes / No
Electric drill/sander	Yes / No	Yes / No
Motorcycle	Yes / No	Yes / No
Motor mower	Yes / No	Yes / No
Power lathe	Yes / No	Yes / No
Snowmobile	Yes / No	Yes / No
Snow blower	Yes / No	Yes / No
Hedge/Tree trimmer	Yes / No	Yes / No
Other specify: _____	Yes / No	Yes / No
Opinion—exposure significant	Yes / No	Yes / No

SECTION 5   SYMPTOMS

a. *Blanching*

   i. Do you ever experience blanching of your fingers?   Yes / No

   ii. When did the fingertip blanching first occur ___ year

             Latent interval _____ years.

   iii. Indicate which digits are affected and distribution:

	RL	RR	RM	RI	RT	LT	LI	LM	LR	LL	Fin.	Th.
Dist.	__	__	__	__	__	__	__	__	__	__	1	4
Mid.	__	__	__	__			__	__	__	__	2	-
Prox.	__	__	__	__	__	__	__	__	__	__	3	5

Score Right _____   Score Left_____   Total_____

   iv. On average, how long does each episode last?_____

   _____

   v. At what time does it occur now—at work?   Yes / No

                   —at home?   Yes / No

   vi. Does any factor (exempli gratia, cold) trigger it? Specify:

   _____

    vii. How often does it occur? daily/weekly/regularly/occasionally

   viii. Does it occur in warm weather?   Yes / No

    ix. Does it affect any of your normal activities?   Yes / No

     x. If yes, specify:_____

_____

    xi. Present state: stationary/improving/deteriorating

b. *Numbness*

     i. Do you ever experience numbness in your fingers?   Yes / No

    ii. Indicate which digits are affected:

   RL RR RM RI   RT   LT LI   LM LR LL

   iii. When did this first occur?_____

_____

    iv. At what time does it occur now—at work?   Yes / No

                        —at home?   Yes / No

                        —at night?   Yes / No

                        —during blanching?   Yes / No

                        —after blanching?   Yes / No

     v. Does any factor (exempli gratia, cold) trigger it? Specify:_____

_____

    vi. How often does it occur? daily/weekly/regularly/occasionally

                        intermittent/persistent

   vii. Does it occur in warm weather?   Yes / No

   viii. Does it affect any of your normal activities?   Yes / No

     x. If yes, specify:_____

_____

    ix. Do you have any difficulty handling small objects   Yes / No

        If yes, specify:_____

_____

    xi. Present state: stationary/improving/deteriorating

c. *Tingling* (This does not refer to transient tingling in the fingers immediately after using vibrating tools)

    i. Do you ever experience tingling in your fingers?   Yes / No

    ii. Indicate which digits are affected:

        RL   RR   RM   RI   RT   LT   LI   LM   LR   LL

    iii. When did this first occur?_____

    iv. At what time does it occur now—at work?   Yes / No
                         —at home?   Yes / No
                         —at night?   Yes / No
                         —after blanching?   Yes / No

    v. Does any factor (for exempli gratia, cold) trigger it? Specify:_____

_____

    vi. How often does it occur?   daily/weekly/regularly/occasionally

    vii. Does it occur in warm weather?   Yes / No

    viii. Does it affect any of your normal activities?   Yes / No

    ix. If yes, specify:_____

_____

    x. Present state: stationary/improving/deteriorating

d. *Other*

    i. Do your fingers ever turn blue (cyanosis)?   Yes / No

    ii. Have you had any trophic changes? Specify:_____ Yes / No

_____

e. *Neuromuscular*

    i. Do you have any difficulty with fine movements of your fingers? Yes / No

       Specify:_____

_____

    ii. Do you have any weakness in the hands or arms? Specify: Yes / No

_____

iii. Do you have any other symptoms relating to the hands or arms?   Yes / No

  Specify:_____

HISTORY CONCLUSION

  Stockholm Grading (Vascular) _____

  Stockholm Grading (Sensorineural) _____

PROTECTIVE PRACTICE

a. At work_____

  Gloves:_____

  Clothing: _____

b. Away from work (extra precautions):_____

  _____

OPINION:

SECTION 6   CLINICAL ASSESSMENT

Hands, muscle and soft tissue (describe) _____

_____

	Left	*Right*
Scars	_____	_____
Callosities	_____	_____
Dupuytren's contracture	_____	_____
Muscle wasting	_____	_____
Other findings:	_____	_____

VASCULAR

	Left	Right
Brachial pulse	good/poor/absent	good/poor/absent
Radial pulse	good/poor/absent	good/poor/absent
Ulnar pulse	good/poor/absent	good/poor/absent
Adson's test	−ve/+ve	−ve/+ve

Blood pressure R.____/____mmHg   sitting/lying/standing

L.____/____mmHg

Pulse rate _____per minute

Hand Circulation

	Left	Right
Finger temperature	cool/warm	cool/warm
Lewis-Prusik test	normal/abnormal	normal/abnormal
Allen's test—Ulnar (seconds)	____ normal/abnormal	____ normal/abnormal
—Radial	____ normal/abnormal	____ normal/abnormal

Cyanosis present?
(if so, describe area) _____

Carpal Tunnel Syndrome

	Left	Right
Tinel's test	−ve/+ve	−ve/+ve
Phalen's test	−ve/+ve	−ve/+ve

Skin Sensitivity

	Depth Sense		Two Point	
	Left	Right	Left	Right
Index	____	____	____	____
Middle	____	____	____	____
Ring	____	____	____	____
Little	____	____	____	____

Grip Strength   Left____Kg   Right____Kg

Manipulative Dexterity (comment on abnormality):

Significant
_____Yes   _____No

NEUROLOGICAL

Arm Reflexes

	Left			Right		
	Absent	Present	Hyper.	Absent	Present	Hyper.
Radial	___	___	___	___	___	___
Bicipital	___	___	___	___	___	___
Tricipital	___	___	___	___	___	___

HAND-ARM VIBRATION SYNDROME—LABORATORY TESTS PERFORMED

a. Audiometry — Yes / No
b. Vibrometer — Yes / No
c. Current perception threshold (CPT) — Yes / No
d. Thermal detection threshold — Yes / No
e. Nerve conduction — Yes / No
f. Doppler   arms — Yes / No
        legs — Yes / No
g. Plethysmography   fingers — Yes / No
        toes — Yes / No
h. Finger systolic pressure
    at 30°C — Yes / No
    at 10°C — Yes / No
    at 10°C + cold blanket — Yes / No
i. Digit temperature test at 21°C room temperature
    (blanket at 45°C; Water bath at 10°C) — Yes / No
j. Urinalysis — Yes / No
k. Blood Tests — Yes / No
    Cell count + differential
    E.S.R.
    Cryoglobulins
    Antinuclear and rheumatoid factors
    Haem. Immunoelectrophoresis
    Uric Acid
l. X-ray Hands/Wrist — Yes / No
    Elbows — Yes / No
    Neck — Yes / No

DIAGNOSTIC GRADING

Stockholm: Vascular_____   Sensorineural_____

Hand-Arm Vibration Syndrome

Health Surveillance Follow-Up Assessment

Date___ / ___ / ____

Last Name _____First Name_____

Date of last assessment ____/____ /____

SECTION 1

a. Any change of address or Physician details?   Yes / No

If yes, specify:_____

_____

b. Any change in duties?   Yes / No

If yes, new job title _____

Description of work_____

Tools used _____

Approximate time exposed to vibration: hours per week _____

weeks per year _____

No. of years _____

Date changed job ____/____ /____

213

c. Any change in leisure exposure to vibration?   Yes / No

If yes, specify: _____

_____

d. Any change in health status, illness or injury?   Yes / No

If yes, specify: _____

_____

e. Any change in medication?   Yes / No

If yes, specify: _____

_____

f. Any change in smoking pattern?   Yes / No

If yes, specify: _____

_____

g. Any change in alcohol consumption?   Yes / No

If yes, specify: _____

_____

h. Any change in hobbies?   Yes / No

If yes, specify: _____

_____

SECTION 2—Symptoms

SECTION 3—Clinical assessment as for initial assessment

OPINION:

Appendix 2

Workplace Tool Assessment CheckList

TOOL DESCRIPTION

Date ___ / ___ / ____

Type (exempli gratia, drill, sander, trimmer): _____

Make _____ Model _____ Serial number: _____,

Brief description _____.

_____

_____

Last serviced (date) _____ General condition _____

Type of power: Electrical _____ Gasoline _____

Pneumatic (PSI operating) _____ Other_____

Condition of accessories (exempli gratia, bits, wheels, chisels, as used with tool):

_____

Weight _____ Supply Voltage (110/120) _____ RPM _____
(Probable dominant frequency = RPM divided by 60)
Torque: High/moderate/low.   Type of clutch: Cut-off/slip/N.A

215

TOOL USAGE

The tool is:—Hand held (one or both): _____   Yes / No
       —Floor mounted   Yes / No
       —Table mounted   Yes / No
       —Suspended   Yes / No
       —Others (specify):   Yes / No

Actual operating time per day: Hrs. _____Minutes_____

Actual operating time per week: Hrs. _____Minutes_____

Actual operating days per year:_____
Time study confirmation of vibration contact time: Yes / No
Tool used:—Continuously   Yes / No
       —Intermittently (with vibration free work periods) Yes / No
       —Daily/weekly/occasionally.

Type of work piece (specify, exempli gratia, steel, plastic, wood): _____
Usual working environment:—Indoor/outdoor.
                         —Cold/warm/hot.

TOOL VIBRATION MEASUREMENT DATA

Acceleration
Weighted a_x_____ m/sec² Unweighted a_x_____m/sec²
              a_y_____ m/sec² a_y_____m/sec²
              a_z_____ m/sec² a_z_____m/sec²
Location and mounting of accelerometer (specify exempli gratia, hand-arm attachment, stud mounting, cement mounting):

_____

Measurement procedure:—Direct measurement   Yes / No
                       —Analysis of tape recorded signals   Yes / No
Equipment used for measurement/analysis

Make _____ Model _____ Serial No. _____
Diagram of set-up (If not direct measurement):

Task performed during measurement:_____

Name of worker operating the tool: _____

VIBRATION EXPOSURE EVALUATION

HAV standard(s) being used for evaluation: _____
Conclusion: —Percentile risk:_____%
        —Standard exceeded: Yes / No
        —Specify further action required (exempli gratia, further measure-
           ments, tool modification, restriction on use of tool):

_____

_____

_____

                    Signed (Investigator)

Glossary

This vocabulary defines terms used with a specialized meaning in this book, in the literature, and in standards pertaining to human exposure to vibration. The reader is referred to appropriate dictionaries for definitions of medical, engineering, or other terms not specific to this field. Abbreviations in common use in human vibration-exposure research, measurement, and related clinical practice are included. Additional terminology used in biodynamics, which has received international standardization, is to be found in international standards ISO 2631-1978, ISO 5349-1986, and ISO 5805-1981.

Acceleration: The rate of change of velocity or speed.
Accelerometer: A transducer that measures acceleration.
Abbreviations:
  ACGIH: American Conference of Government Industrial Hygienists.
  ANSI: American National Standards Institute.
  BSI: British Standards Institution.
  CMI: Cornell Medical Index.
  CTD: Cumulative trauma disorder.
  CTS: Carpal tunnel syndrome.
  DHSS: Department of Health & Social Security Office, U.K.
  EL: Exposure limit.
  EEG: Electroencephalogram.
  EMG: Electromyogram.
  FDP: Fatigue decreased proficiency.
  FSBP: Finger systolic blood pressure.
  HAV: Hand-arm vibration (syn: HTV).
  HAVS: Hand-arm vibration syndrome.
  HSE: Health and Safety Executive, U.K.
  HTV: Hand-transmitted vibration (syn: HAV).
  ISO: International Organization for Standardization.
  MSI: Motion sickness incidence.
  PRP: Primary Raynaud's phenomenon.

RC: Reduced comfort.

REL: Recommended exposure level.

SRP: Secondary Raynaud's phenomenon.

VWF: Vibration white finger.

WBV: Whole-body vibration.

Amplitude (m): Momentary maximum value of a quantity.

Antivibration (A/V): Material or device to reduce the transfer of vibration from a tool or glove to the hands, or from a structure to the whole body.

Arthrosis: Degeneration in a joint.

Arteriography: X-ray of arteries after the intravascular injection of a radiopaque substance.

Broad-band vibration: Vibration with frequency content of more than one third octave or one octave.

Callus: Area of skin thickened by hypertrophy of the horny layer of the epidermis, caused by friction or pressure.

Conditioning preamplifiers: Electronic amplifiers used with accelerometers to amplify and shape their output characteristics.

Coordinate systems (biodynamic): Since vibration is a vector quantity, the intersection of three mutually perpendicular axes are chosen to perform three linear vibration measurements. The biodynamic or basicentric systems define these measurement points and directions.

Coupling: The ability of vibration to travel across or between multiple structures, (exempli gratia, a vibrating hand-tool and the hand).

Crest factor: The ratio of the peak vibration value to the root-mean-square (rms) value.

Damping: The dissipation of vibration energy by conversion into heat.

Displacement: The distance between the normal resting or equilibrium position of an object and its position at any given time in a vibration cycle.

Electromyography: A graphic record of the electric activity of a muscle either spontaneously or in response to artificial electric stimulation.

Ergonomics: The science of human work and its application to the workers' safety, efficiency, and well-being.

Esthesiometer: Instrument for measuring tactile sensibility.

Frequency: The number of complete cycles occurring in one second. Expressed in hertz (Hz) or cycles per second.

Fourier spectrum analysis: A method for the analysis of vibration frequency components and their relative intensities and phase.

Fundamental: The lowest frequency component in a vibration spectrum.

Gravity or "g": The normal force of gravity on earth. ($1g = 9.81 \text{m/sec}^2$)

Hand-arm vibration: Vibration of the human upper limb.

Harmonic motion: Simple harmonic motion occurs when there is a sinusoidal oscillation at a single frequency. The most commonly encountered motions contain vibration at more than one frequency. In some cases the mixture of frequencies contains harmonics.

Harmonics: Multiples (or overtones) of the fundamental vibration frequency.

Isolation: The reduction of vibration by the intentional separation of mechanical transmission between source and receiver.

Jerk: The rate of change of acceleration with respect to time.

Kinetosis: Motion sickness.

Mechanical impedance: The ratio of vibration force to velocity at the driving or transfer point.

Mechanical vibration: Vibration transmitted to (or affecting) man from the motion or vibration of structures or other sources.

Motion sickness incidence: The percentage of a population succumbing to motion sickness within a specified time.

Octave band: A frequency band whose upper limit is twice the lower one.

One-third octave band: An octave band contains three, one third octave bands of equal width on a log scale.

Paresthesia: Sensation of tingling, prickling, or burning of the skin.

Peak value: The maximum value of the amplitude point in a vibration wave form.

Periodic motion: Reciprocating motion that repeats itself over and over.

Plethysmography: Measurement of volume changes of a blood vessel, usually in peripheral arteries.

Random vibration: Vibration that cannot be predicted for any given instant of time.

Resonance frequency: The vibration frequency or frequencies at which the vibration receiver is optimally coupled (or tuned) to the source, resulting in internal amplification (exacerbation of the impinging vibration).

Root-mean-square (rms): The square root of the mean of the squared vibration values.

Sinusoidal motion: Motion that is a sinusoidal function of time (analogous to a pure tone in acoustics).

Sensorineural: Of or pertaining to sensory nerves.

Somatosensory: Pertaining to bodily sensation.

Temperature spectrum map: A computerized method using a 3-D graphics display to determine the vibration damping characteristics of materials. The horizontal X-axis of the display gives vibration frequency; the vertical Y-axis shows temperature; and the Z-axis shows vibration modes (resonances) of the material under test.

Thermography: A diagnostic technique that records infrared radiation emanating from the body.

Transmissibility: The ratio of vibration output acceleration to input acceleration as a function of frequency. A ratio of one indicates that the vibration entering the system leaves the system unaltered. A ratio less than one indicates that the system is attenuating the input vibration. A ratio greater than one indicates amplification of the input vibration (resonance).

Triaxial vibration measurement: Three mutually perpendicular measurements taken simultaneously at the same point.

Vector: A quantity that is completely determined by its magnitude and direction.

Velocity: The rate of change of displacement with time.

Vibration: Any reciprocating (or oscillatory) motion.

Whole-body vibration (WBV): Vibration of the whole body of a human being.

Index

221

Keinbock's disease, 32, 36, 64. *See also* Bones, lunate

Latent interval, 115, 116
Legal issues:
    avoiding litigation, 195–199
    common law claims, 191–194
    compensation, 187, 189, 194
    degree of impairment, 189, 191
    lawsuits, 188
    State benefit, 189, 190
    United States, 186–189
    United Kingdom, 189
    warnings, 187, 198
Link lengths, 139, 144. *See also* Ergonomic stress factors, posture
Locomotor System, 62–65

Mechanoreceptors:
    Meissner, 12, 13, 15–17
    Merkel cell-neurite, 12, 14, 15, 17
    Pacinian, 12, 13–17
Medical surveillance, 102. *See also* Health
Metacholine, 50, 51
Muscle:
    cell hypertrophy, 51, 52, 54
    function, 64
    power, 35, 64
    smooth muscle cell, 42, 45, 49, 51
    strength, 33, 64. *See also* Grip, force; Tests, grip strength
    weakness (dystrophy), 64, 65
Muscles:
    abductor digiti minimi, 5
    abductor pollicis brevis, 5
    adductor pollicis, 5
    flexor carpi radialis, 35
    flexor digiti minimi, 5
    flexor digitorum profundus, 35
    flexor digitorum sublimis, 35
    flexor pollicis brevis, 5
    flexor pollicis longus, 35
    interrosseous, 5
    lumbrical, 5
    opponens digiti minimi, 5
    opponens pollicis, 5
    palmaris longus, 35

Nerve fibres:

epineural edema, 59
fast-adapting, 15, 16
group A, 11, 12, 17
group A-alpha, 12, 14
group A-beta, 12, 14, 15
group A-delta, 12, 14
group B, 11, 12, 17
group C, 11, 12, 14, 17
slow-adapting, 15, 16
Nerve roots:
    brachial plexus, 7
    cervical distribution, 9
Nerves:
    autonomic, 10, 12, 17
    brachial plexus, 5, 7
    lateral cutaneous, 8
    medial cutaneous, 7, 8
    median, 5, 8, 35, 58, 59, 61, 62
    myelinated, 11, 12, 14, 17
    nonmyelinated, 11, 12, 17
    posterior cutaneous, 7, 8
    radial, 1, 8
    subclavian, 1
    ulnar, 6, 7, 8, 35, 58, 59, 61, 62, 68
Neuropathy:
    diffuse, 54, 58–62
Neuropsychiatric symptoms, 34, 65, 66, 68. *See also* Systemic disease
Nicotine, 57
Nitric oxide, 50
Noise:
    and Vibration, 55
    impulse, 33
Norepinepherine (NE), 48, 56

Obstructive arterial disease, 22, 23
Occupations:
    brush cutters, 107
    caulkers, 105, 109, 110
    chainsaw operators, 106
    chippers, 110
    drillers, 108, 109, 110
    fettlers, 105, 109
    grinders, 110, 111
    motorcycle speedway riders, 107, 113
    platers, 111
    riveters, 105, 109
    stonecutters, 110
Osteoarthritis, 32, 36
Osteoarthrosis, 63, 64